Prayers
OF A PEACEFUL
Warrior

WRITTEN BY
ROBIN K. INGRAM

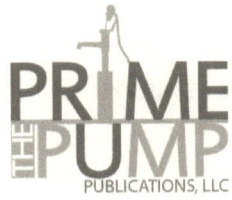

PRAYERS OF A PEACEFUL WARRIOR

Copyright © 2021 by Robin K. Ingram

Cover and page layout by Prime The Pump Publications

All Rights Reserved

Contents and/or cover may not be reproduced in whole or in part in any form without the express written consent of the Publisher.

Scripture quotations marked (NIV) are taken from the Holy Bible, New International Version®, NIV®. Copyright © 1973, 1978, 1984, 2011 by Biblica, Inc.™ Used by permission of Zondervan. All rights reserved worldwide. www.zondervan.com. The "NIV" and "New International Version" are trademarks registered in the United States Patent and Trademark Office by Biblica, Inc.™

Unless otherwise indicated, all Scripture quotations are taken from the Holy Bible, New Living Translation, copyright © 1996, 2004, 2015 by Tyndale House Foundation. Used by permission of Tyndale House Publishers, Carol Stream, Illinois 60188. All rights reserved.

ISBN 978-1-947380-02-8

Library of Congress Control Number: 2021913922

Printed in the United States of America.

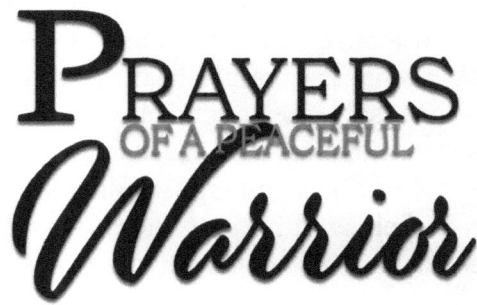

"Prayers of a Peaceful Warrior: Being Anchored to Fulfill Your Purpose speaks to the spirit and soul of mankind. The prayers and teaching instilled in Robin by her mother has produced this wonderful fruitfulness. The prayers and inspirational messages, scriptures and reflections will uplift many across the globe."

>Margaret I.
>Retired Law Enforcement Officer
>*Philadelphia, PA*

"Sometimes it is hard to formulate the right words to put into a simple prayer to our creator. With life being so busy she has been able to perfectly describe and pen a prayer for a warrior's everyday needs. Her passages lend itself perfectly to easy journaling and permanent application. Reading the passages keeps me ever mindful of God's daily presence with us. Thank you for allowing God to use your vessel in writing these powerful passages and prayers."

>Felicia Grant-Hopkins
>Philanthropist
>*Abingdon, MD*

"I love the idea and energy! Prayer is a powerful resource/tool in any given situation...it rebukes the enemy, allows for heavy burdens to be released and it certainly encourages healthy, abundant and graceful outlooks...but everyone isn't super confident in their praying abilities... so a book like this is an excellent idea...especially for those feeling less confident in being able to find powerful healing words...while giving the readers privacy in their sensitive season(s) ... Awesome!....This book will sow healing seeds in many people's lives...Love it! Wonderful."

         Coach Lakia
         YouTuber & Life Coach

Dedication

Being confident of this very thing, that he who has begun a good work in you will perform it until the day of Jesus Christ - Philippians 1:6 (KJV)

In honor of my mother, Carline E. Ingram, our Queen Warrior, faithful servant of God who taught me about the power of prayer. *"Be careful for nothing; but in everything by prayer and supplication with thanksgiving let your requests be made known unto God."* Philippians 4:6 (KJV)

To my Angel Network, *"Each of you should use whatever gift you have received to serve others, as faithful stewards of God's grace in its various forms."* 1 Peter 4:10 (NIV). May God continue to allow us to ascend higher in him.

In loving memory of Pastor James E. Woods II. I honor your legacy. Your purpose was fulfilled. As God's spirit-filled vessel, you helped authors who had a spiritual word from God to find its way to print.

"Commit your way to the Lord." Psalms 37:5a (NIV)

HOW DO YOU APPLY THIS DEVOTIONAL TO YOUR LIFE?

Did you know that prayer is our love language to God? Have you ever wondered, How do I pray and what should I say to God when I pray? Does God hear my prayers? What does having a prayer life look like? Can I truly overcome this trauma, depression and anxiety? Will I be delivered from the heaviness in my heart? Can God help me find and fulfill my purpose?

Using a holistic approach to developing a prayer life, in her own voice, Ms. Robin K. Ingram serves as a guide by your side. She has incorporated a versatile approach to her reflection activities after each prayer, to engage, nurture and address the diverse learning styles of each reader. Prayers of a Peaceful Warrior encourages you to set aside time that is dedicated for your personal reflection and worship. It ignites an authentic relationship with God that ultimately becomes a part of who you are, not just what you do each day. As you progress along the spiritual continuum of development, this devotional provides prayers that enhance a spiritual growth mindset. It also addresses how to maintain a healthy and balanced life in the thoughtfully created self-development reflection activities.

Robin also recommends taking time in nature while connecting with our Creator. She poses intriguing questions that will allow you to reflect, journal, draw, listen to music, view videos, and create and practice positive affirmations.

Throughout the book, you will find stimulating reflection activities that will take you directly to Robin's YouTube channel, ***Angel Network***

HOW DO YOU APPLY THIS DEVOTIONAL TO YOUR LIFE?

Ascension. Using a spiritual foundation, you are given an opportunity to apply what was learned to your life in a meaningful way. With a careful focus on the Word of God, Prayers of a Peaceful Warrior will be a resource in your spiritual war chest that helps to combat distractions of the enemy. This devotional will also help you focus on:

- Maintaining your mental health through mindfulness
- Increasing your faith in God
- Exercising an attitude of gratitude
- Expressing love through prayer
- Learning life lessons of wisdom
- Demonstrating servitude and leadership
- Showing forgiveness & creating unity

In addition to her heartfelt prayers, Robin's personal stories give you a glimpse inside her life of being raised in a Christian home. No matter where you are along your spiritual journey, Robin has a prayer that will comfort you, touch your heart, uplift your spirit and give you encouragement as you use your spiritual gifts to fulfill your purpose.

TABLE OF CONTENTS

Dedication 5
How Do You Apply This Devotional To Your Life? 7

Wellness: Maintaining a Peaceful & Balanced Life Through Prayer

Finding Strength, Psalms 139:23 14
Rest For My Soul, Matthew 11:28-29 15
I Am Never Alone, Romans 8:31 16
Finding Peace, Philippians 4:7 17
God Is By My Side, Zephaniah 3:17 18
There's No Need to Worry, Psalms 27:1 19
A Peaceful Mind, Colossians 3:15 20
Prepared for Spiritual Warfare, Ephesians 6:12 21
God Is My Hope, Psalms 119:114 22
Peace Is a Gift From God, John 14:27 23
God Strengthens Me, Ephesians 3:21 24
God Fortifies Us, Isaiah 40:29 25
Maintaining an Attitude of Gratitude, Philippians 4:8 26
God Gives Us Power Over Our Thoughts, Romans 8:6 27

Prayers on Faithfulness

The Battle Is Already Won, Isaiah 54:17 29
God's Promises Are True, Hebrews 13:8 30
Apply Faith To Your Daily Life, Romans 10:17 31
Delay Is Not Denial, Philippians 2:13 32

Trust In The Lord, Proverbs 3:5-6 33
Surrender To God, Hebrews 11:6.. 34
God Will Fight Our Battles, Exodus 14:14.. 35
Standing On God's Word, Hebrews 11:1 36
Be Strong In The Lord, Ephesians 6:10 37
It Shall Be Well, Romans 8:28 38
God's Grace is Sufficient For Me, 2 Corinthians 12:9............................. 39
Just Pray and Believe, Mark 9:23 40
Be Faithful to God, Psalms 34:8 41

Developing a Prayer Life

God Hears My Prayers, Romans 8:26... 43
Developing a Relationship With Christ, Romans 15:13 44
Guide My Steps, Lord, Psalms 119:11 45
An Intimate Relationship With Christ, 1 Chronicles 16:11 46
Give Me a Pure Heart, Lord, Matthew 6:7 47
Seek God First For Everything, Matthew 6:33 48
The Divine Connection, Psalms 16:11 49
To Be In God's Presence, James 1:13 50
The Holy Spirit Lives In Me, 1 Corinthians 3:16 51
Let Your Light Shine In Me, 1 John 1:5 52
Purify My Spirit, God, Psalms 51:1-2 53
Spending Devoted Time With God, Matthew 6:6................................... 54
Help Me Meditate On You and Not My Mishaps, Joshua 1:8 55
Connecting With the Creator, Romans 1:20 56
His Amazing Grace (The Ultimate Sacrifice), Romans 3:25 57
We Exalt You Jesus!, Isaiah 60:3 58
Let's Walk In God's Light Together, 1 John 5:7 59

Prayers of Comfort

All Things Are Possible With Christ, Philippians 4:13.......................... 61
God's Unfailing Love, Psalms 59:16 62
God Heals Broken Hearts, Psalms 147:3 63
Replenish Our Souls, Jeremiah 31:25 64
God Is Our Refuge, Nahum 1:7 65

Honoring Mom: Our Queen Warrior

Nuggets of Wisdom, Matthew 5:4 67
Life Lessons From Mom, James 1:17.. 68
Memories of Mom 69
I Would Also Like To Share A Personal Story About My Father,
Ronald M. Ingram, Sr. 70
Don't Borrow Any Worry From Tomorrow, Matthew 6:34................ 71

Expressing Gratitude & Love Through Prayer

My Life Is In Your Hands, Jeremiah 29:11 73
Grateful For Forgiveness, Psalms 85:2 74
Grateful To Experience God's Greatness, Habakkuk 2:14 75
Empathy vs. Sympathy, Galatians 6:2 76
Grateful For My Blessings, Matthew 6:19 77
God, Thank You For Being There For Me, 1 Peter 4:16..................... 78
Agape Love, John 13:34 79
Show Kindness and Love, 1 Corinthians 13:1 80
Representing God's Love, Micah 6:8 81
Grateful For God's Presence In My Life, Psalms 23:6 82
Peace That Surpasses All Understanding, Isaiah 54:10 83
Loving Traits of a Christian, Colossians 3:12...................................... 84
Cautiously Use the Power of Your Words, Proverbs 15:1 85
Be a Testament of God's Love, 1 Timothy 2:5 86
Demonstrate Love Everywhere You Go, Zephaniah 2:3 87
Unconditional Love, 1 Corinthians 16:13.. 88
Our Compassionate God, Lamentations 3:22-23 89

Servitude, Leadership & Wisdom

Living a Purpose-Filled Life, Matthew 28:19...................................... 91
Share the Good News, 2 Timothy 2:15 92
I Am God's Spirit-Filled Vessel, 1 Corinthians 10:31 93
Serve With Honor, Warrior, Mark 8:34... 94
Be a Wise Leader, Proverbs 9:10 95
God Gives Us the Wisdom to Lead, John 15:4 96
God Is Our Anchor, James 3:13 97

Remain Teachable, Proverbs 3:7 98
Success Defined Through the Eyes of God, 1 Peter 5:6 99
The Body of Christ; Serving Others, 1 Corinthians 12: 25-27 100
Renewing the Mind, Romans 12:2 101
Foundation of True Knowledge, Proverbs 1:7 102
Serve In a Spirit of Love, Psalms 68:19 103
A Servant's Heart, Matthew 6:3 104
Lessons Learned From God, Philippians 4:9 105
Choose Today Whom You Will Serve, Joshua 24:15 106
Be Kind to One Another and Show Compassion, Galatians 5:13 107
More Like Jesus, Matthew 5:8 108
Persevere Despite Persecution, Luke 6:27-28 109
Guard Your Heart, Proverbs 4:23 110
Be a Beacon of Light, Colossians 4:6 111
Loyalty in Friendships, Proverbs 11:17 112
Grace From Above, Psalms 1:1 113
Where God Leads, I Will Follow, Proverbs 22:6 114

Forgiveness & Unity

Forgive Yourself, Proverbs 27:5 117
Forgive One Another, Ephesians 4:32 118
Love Your Enemies!, Luke 6:35 119
Fully Forgive Others, 2 John 1:6 120
Mold Me, Jesus!, Romans 15:5 121

A Prayer For Our Nation

A Unified Focus For the Kingdom of God, Matthew 18:20 123
A Prayer For Our Nation 124

Notes

Wellness: Maintaining a Peaceful & Balanced Life Through Prayer

Finding Strength

Search Me, O God, And Know My Heart...
PSALMS 139:23 (NIV)

Dear Gracious Heavenly Father,

You are omnipotent. You are omniscient; therefore, there is nothing that I can keep hidden from you. Search my heart, God. Help me to surrender to you and free myself of all the anxious thoughts that may be contaminating my mind and weighing down my heart. You know all about me because you created me. Help me to find strength in my vulnerability. When I am weak, you are strong. Father, please live in my heart and soul each day. Thank you for your mercy, grace and love even when I have fallen short of your grace. You are our gracious God. Please continue to watch over and bless my family and friends. I love you today and always.

In Jesus' name,

Amen

Reflection: Allow self-compassion to free you. Ask God for his help as you deal with anxious thoughts that may arise on your daily walk.

Rest For My Soul

> "Come to me, all you who are weary and burdened, and I will give you rest. Take my yoke upon you and learn from me, for I am gentle and humble in heart, and you will find rest for your souls."
> MATTHEW 11:28-29 (NLT)

Dear Gracious Heavenly Father,

Thank you for this beautiful day that you have made, let us rejoice and be glad in it. Father, thank you for your provision. In this life, we tend to rush from task to task without taking the time to rest. You already have plans for our lives, so instead of us always being in "hurry mode," please help us to just rest in you. In your word, in Matthew 11:28-29, you tell us:

"Come to me, all you who are weary and burdened, and I will give you rest. Take my yoke upon you and learn from me, for I am gentle and humble in heart, and you will find rest for your souls." Help us to cast our cares and burdens on you because you care for us. Thank you, Father, for your love. We trust in your word and promises.

In Jesus' name,

Amen

Reflection: Write down 3 things that are currently causing you unrest. Write each one down on a separate piece of paper. Drop each piece of paper into a small container. Label this box: Your "God's got it" box! Begin to thank God for allowing you to rest in him.

I Am Never Alone

"If God be for us, who can be against us?"
ROMANS 8:31 (KJV)

Dear Gracious Heavenly Father,

You are such an awesome God! You died so that I may be free. When I think about the times in my life when I face challenges, I try my best to not allow myself to get overwhelmed because I know that I am not alone. I walk into the face of adversity with you by my side because in Romans 8:31, I have learned:

"If God be for us, who can be against us?" Therefore I know that the battle is not mine to fight alone. I am more than a conqueror because you are right by my side. I now realize that I must relinquish my concerns to you because you want the very best for me. I thank you for the inheritance that I have in you as your child. Thank you for your love and protection, Father. I give you praise, honor and glory today and forever.

In Jesus' name,

Amen

Reflection: Take a moment to reflect on every answered prayer and every blessing that God has given you as a reminder of who he is in your life.

Finding Peace

And the peace of God, which surpasses all understanding, will guard your hearts and minds through Christ Jesus.
PHILIPPIANS 4:7 (KJV)

Dear Gracious Heavenly Father,

Thank you for this day. Thank you for your mercy and grace. Thank you for your protection. Father, in this life, circumstances will arise that can cause us to feel unsettled. In your word you taught us:

"And the peace of God, which passeth all understanding, shall keep your hearts and minds through Christ Jesus." Help me, Father, to refocus my perspective, to stay focused on you so that my ability to trust in you produces peace that surpasses all understanding. Father, please let your peace fill my life, guard my heart and every aspect of who I am. No matter what goes on around me, allow me to find rest in you and your promises. Please give me the strength to persevere and endure as I stand on your word. Thank you for all the many ways that you have blessed me, my family and our ever growing Angel Network. We honor you today and always.

In Jesus' name,

Amen

Reflection: Think about all of the things that you are grateful for today. Honor your life by thanking God for each one through worship and song.

God Is By My Side

"The Lord your God in your midst, The Mighty One, will save; He will rejoice over you with gladness, He will quiet you with His love, He will rejoice over you with singing."
ZEPHANIAH 3:17 (NIV)

Dear Gracious Heavenly Father,

You are my source and strength. You are my strong tower. I am so grateful to know that you delight in me. In your word you tell us:

"For the Lord your God is living among you. He is a mighty savior. He will take delight in you with gladness. With his love, he will calm all your fears. He will rejoice over you with joyful songs." I realize that there may be times when I am afraid but I know that you are right by my side. You see all things because you are omnipotent. You want to see me succeed and release my mind of a defeated mentality. With you by my side, I will let go of limiting beliefs because your power is limitless. Father, thank you for your protection over my family and friends and the support that they provide. Help us to rest in you as your love washes over us. We honor you today for who you are because you are worthy to be praised!

In Jesus' name,

Amen

> *Reflection: Find a quiet space. Take a moment to close your eyes and take a few deep, cleansing breaths as you place your hands over your heart. Acknowledge in this moment that you are filled with God's love, not fear. Repeat this exercise until you begin to feel centered again. Declare: "God, you have not given me a spirit of fear, but one of power, love and a sound mind."*
> - 2 Timothy 1:7 NKJV

There's No Need to Worry

The Lord is my light and my salvation; whom shall I fear? The Lord is the strength of my life; of whom shall I be afraid?
PSALMS 27:1 (KJV)

Dear Gracious Heavenly Father,

I come before you today with a grateful and courageous heart. Thank you, Father, for listening to my fears and hearing my prayers. In Psalms 27:1, your word says:

"The Lord is my light and my salvation; whom shall I fear? The Lord is the strength of my life; of whom shall I be afraid?" Father, I know that anxiety can present itself in our lives and cause an unsettling feeling, however, you are our fortress. Please help me to remember that you have not given me a fearful spirit. You have filled me with your power which is full of love with a sound mind. When I begin to feel overwhelmed, help me to look to you to provide comfort and stability. Give me the strength to stand with others as I anchor myself in your word and its promises. Thank you for your mercy and grace.

In Jesus' name,

Amen

Reflection: Treat yourself to a special notebook that will be used as your journal. Take some time to write a letter of encouragement to yourself based on
- Psalms 27:1 KJV

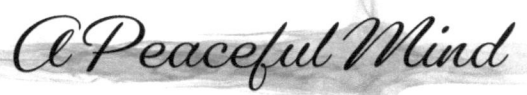

Let the peace of Christ rule in your hearts.
COLOSSIANS 3:15 (NIV)

Dear Gracious Heavenly Father,

I give you praise, honor and glory for who you are in our lives. Father, you are our refuge. You are our Messiah. When the troubles of this world attempt to take up residence in our minds and overshadow our thoughts, you provide us with such peace. In your word you tell us to:

"Let the peace that comes from Christ rule in our hearts. For as members of one body we are called to live in peace." We are to always be thankful. Help us to maintain an attitude of gratitude and rest on your promises because your power is miraculous. You can do anything but fail. Thank you for our beautiful Angel Network and for the community that continues to grow. Bless each individual across the globe and cover them. We give you thanks for all things.

In Jesus' name,

Amen

Reflection: Complete this phrase: Each day, I will maintain an attitude of gratitude by _____.

Prepared for Spiritual Warfare

> For we are not fighting against flesh-and-blood enemies, but against evil rulers and authorities of the unseen world, against mighty powers in this dark world, and against evil spirits in the heavenly places.
> EPHESIANS 6:12 (NLT)

Dear Precious Heavenly Father,

In this life, we are going to face situations where we must truly stand firm on our faith. It's during these times of spiritual warfare where the enemy will tell us lies to distract us from our goals and who we ultimately serve. Father, your omnipresence protects us from seen and unseen harm. I thank you for loving us so much that you place a hedge of protection around us with an army of your angels. Help us to remember that when things go astray, we must pray and stay rooted and grounded in your word as we battle against the evil spirits of this dark world. Please continue to mold us into the faithful warrior that you would have us to be, who possess a willingness to exalt you above all else. We honor you today and forever more.

In Jesus' name,

Amen

Reflection: Maintaining a healthy mind is a key component of wellness. Create a positive affirmation that speaks to the warrior in you.

WELLNESS: MAINTAINING A PEACEFUL & BALANCED LIFE THROUGH PRAYER

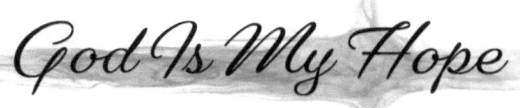

You are my refuge and my shield; your word is my source of hope.
PSALMS 119:114 (NLT)

Dear Heavenly Father,

Your word is hope. Your word is true.

Psalms 119:114 tells us that: *You are my refuge and my shield; your word is my source of hope. Help me to meditate on your word day and night so that my spirit may be peaceful.* Thank you for giving me honorable teachers of your word so that I can learn more and more about you and apply it to my life and spiritual journey. It brings me great comfort when I am strengthened and encouraged by a scripture that helps me to cope in my time of need. Thank you, God, for consistently loving me and for always being by my side. I will forever give your name glory and honor.

In Jesus' name,

Amen

Reflection: Complete this phrase. Thank you Jesus for your love, I will honor you in my life by _____.

Peace Is a Gift From God

> "I am leaving you with a gift—peace of mind and heart. And the peace I give is a gift the world cannot give. So don't be troubled or afraid."
> JOHN 14:27 (NLT)

Dear Gracious Heavenly Father,

Thank you for the gift of your everlasting peace. It is a peace that only you can give and it is not of this world. Help me to rest and abide in the peace that you provide. Knowing you, Father, does not mean that our lives are free of trouble, anxiety or fear. Having the gift of your peace means that we know you will never leave us and that your presence in our lives is constant. What a beautiful blessing! Thank you for teaching me, Father, to have a calm confidence in you and to put my faith in you regardless of the circumstances that may arise. I will rest in your loving arms and cherish the gift of your peace. Please continue to reign over my life and be the steady anchor that I need in the midst of every storm. I honor you today and always.

In Jesus' name,

Amen

Reflection: Today, focus your attention on things that are happening in the present moment. Be mindful of how your attention may get distracted and gently bring it back to the present moment.

God Strengthens Me

To Him be glory in the church by Christ Jesus to all generations, forever and ever. Amen.
EPHESIANS 3:21 (NLT)

Dear Gracious Heavenly Father,

You are AMAZING! You are our King! I magnify your name because you are worthy to be praised! Father, in your word you said that I can do all things through Christ that strengthens me. I know this because there are times when I am completely exhausted, overwhelmed or have a heavy heart and you give me the strength that I need to persevere. Because your power is within me, I can confidently stand on your word that tells me: Now all glory to God, who is able, through his mighty power at work within us, to accomplish infinitely more than we might ask or think. Glory to him in the church and in Christ Jesus through all generations forever and ever! Help me to continue to look to you to do a great work in my life as I strive to uplift others for your glory. I honor you today for reigning over my life. Please bless and cover my family.

In Jesus' name,

Amen

Reflection: If it doesn't challenge you, it won't change you. What are the areas in your life that you need God to help you change?

ROBIN K. INGRAM

God Fortifies Us

He gives power to the weak and strength to the powerless.
ISAIAH **40:29** (NLT)

Dear Gracious Heavenly Father,

Thank you for this beautiful day! We live in a complicated world that often causes us to feel weighed down, overwhelmed and ultimately, stressed and exhausted. I am grateful for knowing that we can find rest in you because you have taught us in your word to:

Come unto you all ye that are heavy laden and you will give us rest. When we are feeling weak, this scripture reminds us of your limitless strength that you will breathe into us. We are not alone. We are more than conquerors in you, Father. Help us to always look to you to be fortified so that we may carry out your will. Thank you for your unconditional love and patience for us each day.

In Jesus' name,

Amen

Reflection: Being courageous over our fears can be challenging. Create 3 affirmations that confirm your knowledge of being a conqueror in Christ. Post these affirmations where you can readily access them and recite them as a part of your daily routine. For example: I am a strong warrior and I am the master over my fear.

Maintaining an Attitude of Gratitude

And now, dear brothers and sisters, one final thing. Fix your thoughts on what is true, and honorable, and right, and pure, and lovely, and admirable. Think about things that are excellent and worthy of praise.
PHILIPPIANS 4:8 (NLT)

Dear Heavenly Father,

I come before you today thanking you for your mercy and grace. I come before you with a humble heart and servant hands thanking you for giving me another opportunity to dwell here on Earth to sing your praises. Father, when we become overwhelmed with the various things that weigh us down, it distracts us from being able to focus on you and hear from you. You have taught us in your word:

"To think on whatsoever things are lovely, pure, honest and of good report..." When we think about these things, it helps us to maintain an attitude of gratitude for all that we have and for all that you have done for us. Thank you for being our Messiah as you continuously watch over and protect us. I pray a special prayer of healing for all those in need of a touch from you today. You are our Jehovah Rapha, our God that heals. We stand on your word and believe in your promises. We give you praise, honor and glory.

In Jesus' name,

Amen

Reflection: Name something that you would like to heal from and begin thanking God for your restoration and deliverance today.

God Gives Us Power Over Our Thoughts

The mind governed by the flesh is death, but the mind governed by the Spirit is life and peace.
ROMANS 8:6 (NIV)

Dear Gracious Heavenly Father,

It's so sweet to know and love you. I thank you for another opportunity to glorify your name and your presence in my life. Father, you taught us to think on whatsoever things are lovely and of good report. It is so easy to get distracted by what is going on all around us in this world and in our daily lives, however, if we focus on you, and look to you for guidance, our lives will have peace. Believing in you gives us such hope that when we pray, we can have confidence in knowing that we can take down those strongholds over our thoughts because of your awesome power! Thank you for your continued patience with us even when we take a path that you did not ordain. You are always right there to correct and forgive us. As we begin a new week, please help us to put you first and follow you along the path that you have designed for our lives.

In Jesus' name,

Amen

Reflection: Reflect on your short-term goals. Have you placed them before the Lord for guidance? Write them down and include them in your daily prayers.

Prayers on Faithfulness

ROBIN K. INGRAM

The Battle Is Already Won

No weapon formed against us shall prosper.
ISAIAH **54:17** (KJV)

Dear Gracious Heavenly Father,

I give you praise, honor and glory, for you are the ruler of the Earth. Just when I think I cannot go on, you remind me that the battle is already won because the war belongs to you. Isaiah 54:17 reminds us that:

"No weapon formed against us shall prosper." Help me, Father, to rise up against the adversity that we face which comes from spiritual forces of evil. Strengthen me to take heart because I know you have overcome the world. Help me to remember that the challenges that I may face are simply the attack on the Holy Spirit which resides in me. Please fortify me with your power and help me to be confident in my faith in you, regardless of the circumstances. You are sovereign. I honor you today for all of my many blessings and how you reign over my life with such love and protection. Please continue to guide me through your light.

In Jesus' name,

Amen

Reflection: Be content with all that you have by practicing gratitude.

PRAYERS ON FAITHFULNESS

God's Promises Are True

*Jesus Christ, the same yesterday,
and today, and forever*
HEBREWS 13:8 (NLT)

Dear Precious Heavenly Father,

You are the living water. Your love for us remains constant. In Hebrews 13:8, your word teaches us that:

"You are the same yesterday, and today, and forever," which means that we can have confidence in knowing that your promises to us will be fulfilled. Although circumstances all around us may indicate that things are falling apart, you have a specific plan for us. Your plan includes providing us with direction, comfort and peace. Please strengthen us, Father, and remind us to look to you for consistent guidance and unconditional love. We honor you today and worship your Holy Name.

In Jesus' name,

Amen

Reflection: Think about this statement. Do not allow your character to change based on your current conditions. What does this mean to you?

Apply Faith To Your Daily Life

*So faith comes from hearing, that is, hearing the
Good News about Christ.*
ROMANS 10:17 (NLT)

Dear Gracious Heavenly Father,

Your word has taught me that without faith it is impossible to please you. There have been many situations in my life when I really needed to exercise my faith in you. I needed to understand that the trials that I faced would ultimately produce more capacity for strength, while my faith in you helped me to persevere and get through my trials. In Romans 10:17, we learn:

"So faith comes from hearing, that is, hearing the Good News about Christ." Now that praying daily, reading your word and applying it to my life is how I exercise my faith, I share that good news with those around me. Father, help me to continue to share your message of faith by demonstrating how you have always shown up for me. Thank you for your many blessings. You will always be sovereign.

In Jesus' name,

Amen

Reflection: Take a moment to reflect on the ways that God shows up for you in your life.

PRAYERS ON FAITHFULNESS

Delay Is Not Denial

For it is God which worketh in you both to will and to do of his good pleasure.
PHILIPPIANS 2:13 (KJV)

Dear Precious Heavenly Father,

I thank you for your mercy and grace. When I think about my life and where I could have been if it was not for your grace protecting me, I am eternally grateful. Just when I thought things were coming "unraveled" in my life, you were putting together a solid plan for my future. You have taught me, Father, in Philippians 2:13:

"For it is God which worketh in you both to will and to do of his good pleasure." Now, I practice patience and exercise faith as I put my trust in you. I no longer confuse delay with denial. I recognize that you are always right by my side, working things out on my behalf. Help me to believe in the power of yet and stand on your promises. The desires of my heart may not be fulfilled yet, however that does not mean that you are not creating a plan just for me. Strengthen me, Father, to carry out the plan that you have designed for me to fulfill in a way that will honor and glorify you. Please continue to bless all those who are connected across the globe, my family and friends.

In Jesus' name,

Amen

Reflection: Click/Copy the link to view my YouTube video, entitled "God's Promises and the Power of Yet." https://youtu.be/NSXE0DbbA0k

Trust In The Lord

Trust in the Lord with all thine heart; and lean not unto thine own understanding. In all thy ways acknowledge him, and he shall direct thy paths.
PROVERBS 3:5-6 (KJV)

Dear Gracious Heavenly Father,

In you will I put my trust. I give you praise, honor and glory for this beautiful day. I thank you, Father, for bringing me to this time in my life. Your desire is for me to totally surrender to you, not just in some things but ALL. In Proverbs 3:5-6, you teach us:

"Trust in the Lord with all thine heart; and lean not unto thine own understanding. In all thy ways acknowledge him, and he shall direct thy paths." Therefore, I will look to you, Father, for guidance and direction for my life. Help me to honor you by putting you first in all that I do. Please keep my mind focused so that I may follow the path that you have created for me. Give me the strength to trust you wholeheartedly without wavering. Thank you for being so patient with me and loving me unconditionally, even when I have gone against your will. Please continue to bless me as I put my trust in you.

In Jesus' name,

Amen

Reflection: If you believe that you are fearfully and wonderfully made, what are you trusting God to do in your life?

PRAYERS ON FAITHFULNESS

Surrender To God

And it is impossible to please God without faith.
HEBREWS 11:6 (NLT)

Dear Gracious Heavenly Father,

Hebrews 11:6 says:

"And it is impossible to please God without faith. Anyone who wants to come to Him must believe that God exists and that He rewards those who sincerely seek Him." Father, there are heavy rocks lying in my path right now, however, I decided to put all of my trust in you. This scripture is not always easy to follow because we must surrender to your will without inserting ourselves into the situation. Father, please strengthen me when the circumstances become difficult and help me to exercise my faith in a consistent way. You said that you would never leave me nor forsake me and I am so grateful for your provision and favor over my life. I feel your presence each day on my daily walk. I am also blessed to experience your unconditional love. You are always with me and that is why I will continue to put my faith in you. I love you, Lord with all my heart.

In Jesus' name,

Amen

Reflection: Go out for a nature walk. Find 3 pebbles. Those pebbles will represent the issues that are currently weighing you down. Walk to the nearest body of water and toss those pebbles in the water as you mentally and emotionally release those burdens unto God.

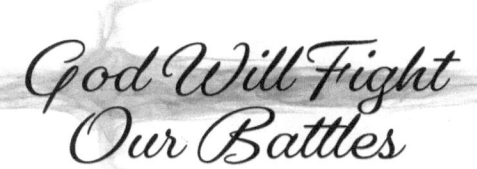

God Will Fight Our Battles

*The Lord shall fight for you,
and ye shall hold your peace.*
EXODUS 14:14 (KJV)

Dear Gracious Heavenly Father,

Thank you, Lord, for this beautiful day. Thank you for protecting us as we rested overnight. In this life, at times, situations can be overwhelming for us to handle on our own. I am grateful for your word in Exodus 14:14 because you tell us:

"The Lord shall fight for you, and ye shall hold your peace." When we are facing difficulties, help us to rest in knowing that you will never leave us nor forsake us. Your power is mighty and you delight in our weakness because in you, we are strong. Help us, Father, to think on whatsoever things are lovely, pure and of good report. Strengthen us and provide comfort so that we can just be still to hear you. You will fight for us, so please help us to trust in you. Please bless every dear heart across the globe today. Thank you for who you are in our lives.

In Jesus' name,

Amen

Reflection: Reflect about positive things in your life and use those thoughts to maintain a peaceful mindset.

Standing On God's Word

*Faith shows the reality of what we hope for;
it is the evidence of things we cannot see.*
HEBREWS 11:1 (NLT)

Dear Gracious Heavenly Father,

Faith is such a precious gift. I thank you for teaching us its meaning in Hebrews 11:1. It reads:

"Faith shows the reality of what we hope for; it is the evidence of things we cannot see." I have learned that it takes spiritual maturity and strength to stand on your word and walk in assurance that you will fulfill your promises. It can be so challenging to maintain our faith because we cannot see the road ahead. Along my spiritual journey, Father, you have shown up for me in ways that I could not ever imagine. It was necessary for me to believe in your word until I saw the evidence of my answered prayers. You have never failed me. You are always with me and I will continue to stand on your word with unwavering faith in you. Thank you for your protection, mercy and love.

In Jesus' name,

Amen

Reflection: Describe what unwavering faith looks like and sounds like in your life?

Be Strong In The Lord

Be strong in the Lord and in the strength of his might.
EPHESIANS 6:10 (KJV)

Dear Gracious Heavenly Father,

I come humbly before you thanking you today because you are my source and strength. I realize, Father, that there will be difficult times that arise in my life, however, in Ephesians 6:10, you remind us:

"Finally, my brethren, be strong in the Lord, and in the power of his might." I am so grateful that I can confidently come to you and know that my strength lies in you. I believe in your power. I declare today that I am strong because you are strong and I will step boldly into the plans you have for my life. I honor you today, for you are my mighty savior. Thank you for reigning over our lives. I give you praise, honor and glory forever.

In Jesus' name,

Amen

Reflection: Create a vision board. Before you begin, pray and ask God for guidance for the direction of your life. Gather all of your craft materials, i.e., magazines, photos, markers, glue, scissors. Upon completion, hold your vision board up to heaven and thank God for reigning over your life as you use the word of God and your vision board as a "navigation tool" for your life.

PRAYERS ON FAITHFULNESS

It Shall Be Well

And we know that all things work together for good to those that love God, to those who are the called according to his purpose.
ROMANS 8:28 (KJV)

Dear Gracious Heavenly Father,

I come before you today thanking you for your many blessings that you see fit to bestow upon me. I give you praise, honor and glory for the universe that you created and all that dwells therein. Help me, Father, to align my life according to the purpose and path that you have designed just for me. In Romans 8:28, you teach us that:

"All things work for the good of those who love him, who have been called according to his purpose." I am so grateful that you reign over my life and although darkness exists in this world, you are our light. We honor you today and continue to give you praise. Thank you for watching over my family, friends and ever-growing Angel Network community.

In Jesus' name,

Amen

Reflection: It's time to count your blessings!! Write down the word BLESSINGS vertically on a piece of paper. Brainstorm words or phrases that describe your blessings. Place your words or phrases on the lines that begin with the same letters.

God's Grace is Sufficient For Me

> "My grace is sufficient for you, for My strength is made perfect in weakness." Therefore most gladly I will rather boast in my infirmities, that the power of Christ may rest upon me.
> 2 CORINTHIANS 12:9 (NIV)

Dear Precious Heavenly Father,

I give you praise, honor and glory, for you are our God. You are omniscient. There have been so many times when I wondered:

How will I make it?

Will I ever feel better?

Can this situation get resolved?

Who is going to help me with this problem?

Then I am reminded of your word and one of my favorite scriptures, where you tell us that:

"My grace is all you need. My power works best in weakness." So now I am glad to boast about my weaknesses, so that the power of Christ can work through me. Time and time again you have shown up for me and been my refuge and strength in my weakness. I am so grateful that when I cried out to you, my prayers were heard and answered. Thank you for your grace, for it is sufficient for me.

In Jesus' name,

Amen

Reflection: What will you believe God for today?

Just Pray and Believe

> "What do you mean, 'If I can'?" Jesus asked. "Anything is possible if a person believes."
> MARK 9:23 (NLT)

Dear Gracious Heavenly Father,

I come before you today with a spirit of humility and gratitude. I thank you for hearing my prayers. Father, thank you for teaching me how important it is to have faith in you and remain confident in what you can and will do, if I just believe. Help me to understand that sometimes prayers will be answered and the outcome may not be what I may have expected, however, your plans for me are what I will follow. For your ways are not our ways and your thoughts are not our thoughts but your path is a righteous one. Thank you for your sacrifice, guidance and love. Thank you for the prayer warriors in my life and in the Angel Network. Bless each one and strengthen them. Please continue to watch over my family and friends. Keep them safe from harm. We honor you today and always.

In Jesus' name,

Amen

Reflection: List 2 ways that you can demonstrate your belief in God's plan for your life.

ROBIN K. INGRAM

Be Faithful to God

Taste and see that the Lord is good. Oh, the joys of those who take refuge in him!
PSALMS 34:8 (NLT)

Dear Gracious Heavenly Father,

What a blessing it is to know you and trust in you! When the troubles of this world begin to mount, it can really be overwhelming. You have taught us in your word how we are to come to you as our refuge and strength. You told us to be like a tree planted by the rivers of water. In your word you said:

"Blessed is the one who trusts in the Lord, whose confidence is in him. They will be like a tree planted by the water that sends out its roots by the stream. It does not fear when heat comes; its leaves are always green. It has no worries in a year of drought and never fails to bear fruit." Father, you want us to remember that when we are confident in you, there is no lack. If we stay faithful and steadfast, we will feel your presence all around us and never be without. Thank you for being our protection and for loving us first. We are grateful for your love and provision as you continuously watch over us. We will honor you today and always.

In Jesus' name,

Amen

Reflection: Describe what you hope to gain by allowing God into your life.

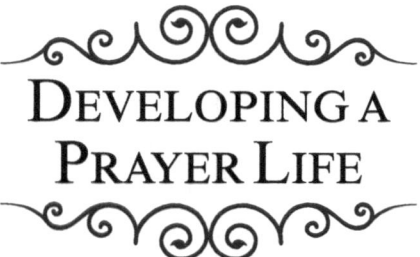

Developing a Prayer Life

ROBIN K. INGRAM

God Hears My Prayers

The Spirit helps us in our weakness.
ROMANS 8:26 (NIV)

Dear Gracious Heavenly Father,

I come humbly before you today with a thankful heart. I am thankful today because I have an opportunity to communicate with you through the Holy Spirit. Having a personal and intimate relationship with you is priceless. It cannot be replaced. Sometimes in prayer, I may lack the ability to know what to say, however, you know my heart and you know my needs. I will continue to cast all of my cares on you because you care for me. Sometimes I may have to just moan and allow the Holy Spirit to intercede on my behalf. Thank you for being such a loving Father, for hearing my prayers and for comforting me. I give you praise honor and glory today for who you are in our lives.

In Jesus' name,

Amen

> *Reflection: Designate a special place in your home as your prayer room. What do you want the room to look and feel like? Invite God into your life and allow him to dwell in all the spaces that you occupy by praying in every area of your home.*

Developing a Relationship With Christ

Now may the God of hope fill you with all joy and peace in believing that you may abound in hope by the power of the Holy Spirit.
ROMANS 15:13 (KJV)

Dear Gracious Heavenly Father,

I give you praise, honor and glory because you are the God of hope. My relationship with you has taught me that although we live in a world full of uncertainty, your desire is for us to trust in you because in your word you said that you are the source of hope, you will fill us completely with joy and peace because we trust in you. Then we will overflow with confident hope through the power of the Holy Spirit. Having you as our guide is such a blessing because you serve as our beacon of light. Help us to remember from whom our blessings flow so that our focus is on our worship and not things. Things are temporary but your love is everlasting! Father, please help us to trust you wholeheartedly and be encouraged by living in expectation of your amazing power. We bless your name forever.

In Jesus' name,

Amen

Reflection: Think back to where you were 6 months ago. On your calendar, jot down what you have accomplished thus far. Write down 3 goals that you would like to accomplish by the end of this year.

ROBIN K. INGRAM

Guide My Steps, Lord

I have hidden your word in my heart so that I might not sin against you.
PSALMS 119:11 (NLT)

Dear Gracious Heavenly Father,

Thank you for this day. Thank you for another opportunity to be in your presence. Father, there are times when we need direction from you. We need to know the right path to take along our journey. This is why I am grateful for your word. It is a lamp unto my feet and a light unto my path. You desire for us to hide your word in our hearts, make it a part of our thought process, so that we do not hurt your heart. You are so merciful to us as you watch over and protect us each day. Thank you, Father. Help us to spend time with you and in your word so that we become closer to you. I honor you for continuing to bless us in so many ways.

In Jesus' name,

Amen

Reflection: Look at your schedule and designate a specific time that you will dedicate daily to your devotional time with God.

DEVELOPING A PRAYER LIFE

An Intimate Relationship With Christ

Search for the LORD and for his strength; continually seek him.
1 CHRONICLES 16:11 (NLT)

Dear Gracious Heavenly Father,

I come before you with you with a humble heart asking you to forgive me for my sins. I am so grateful for the gift of your grace and the ability to come to you through prayer. Thank you for teaching me to seek you first, above all else. In 1 Chronicles 16:11, it teaches us:

"Search for the Lord and for his strength; continually seek him." Help me to spend intentional time with you in prayer in order to accept the plans and design that you have for my life. Thank you for filling me with your wisdom by seeking you first for guidance and direction for my life. I am so grateful for your steady forgiveness and love for me. I will continue to put you first. Thank you for continuing to bless and cover my family and friends.

In Jesus' name,

Amen

Reflection: Examine your commitments. Have you made time to speak with God today?

Give Me a Pure Heart, Lord

> "When we pray, don't babble on and on as the Gentiles do. They think their prayers are answered merely by repeating their words again and again."
> **Matthew 6:7 (NLT)**

Dear Precious Heavenly Father,

I come before you today with a humble heart thanking you for the gift of prayer. In Matthew 6:7 you taught us:

"When we pray, don't babble on and on as the Gentiles do. They think their prayers are answered merely by repeating their words again and again." Don't be like them, for your Father knows exactly what you need even before you ask him! Help me to remember that you are omniscient and therefore you already know what is on my heart. Mold me to develop and maintain an intimate prayer life with you that allows me to have dedicated time with you. Search my heart, Father, to make sure that it is pure when I come before you to pray. Thank you for your unconditional love and protection over us all. Please continue to guide us on our journey as we prioritize you in our lives.

In Jesus' name,

Amen

Reflection: **When you spend time with God, describe how it feels to be in his presence.**

Seek God First For Everything

> "Seek the Kingdom of God above all else, and live righteously, and he will give you everything you need."
>
> MATTHEW 6:33 (NLT)

Dear Gracious Heavenly Father,

Serving you, Father, is not just about singing a worship song. It is about choosing to make room for you in our lives where you are a priority. Matthew 6:33 teaches us to:

"Seek the Kingdom of God above all else, and live righteously, and he will give you everything you need." If we seek you first and do your will, I am so grateful that in you, there is no lack. We are fully covered under your will. I will continue to make you the priority in my life above all else and pray for guidance as you order my steps. Please help me to see things the way that you see things so that I may love others how you love us. Fill me with your loving kindness to share your spirit with others.

In Jesus' name,

Amen

Reflection: Using your senses, look around and identify 3 or more things that you are grateful for that we often take for granted.

The Divine Connection

> You will show me the way of life, granting me the
> joy of your presence and the pleasures of living
> with you forever.
> **Psalms 16:11 (NLT)**

Dear Gracious Heavenly Father,

I give you praise, honor and glory for reigning over my life. In Psalms 16:11, you tell us that:

"You will show me the way of life, granting me the joy of your presence and the pleasures of living with you forever." I know that you will never leave me nor forsake me. Father, developing a true, divine connection with you is what you desire for me because you have designed this path that leads to a full life. Please help me remember that being in your presence blesses my life. Help me to appreciate all of the blessings that you bestow upon me each day. You are a merciful God. I will praise your name forever.

In Jesus' name,

Amen

Reflection: If you could describe your divine connection with God to a friend, what would you share about your experience?

To Be In God's Presence

Let no one say when he is tempted, "I am tempted by God"; for God cannot be tempted by evil, nor does He Himself tempt anyone.
JAMES 1:13 (NIV)

Dear Heavenly Father,

Thank you for this beautiful day! Thank you for reigning over my life. Father, as we make decisions in our lives, please help us to acknowledge you in all of our ways so that you can direct our path. Father, your desire is for us to live full lives of peace and joy and to prosper. This does not mean, however, that our lives will be void of trials, disappointments and challenges that may feel draining at times. It is in these times when we must find strength to persevere and resist the temptation that the enemy attempts to introduce into our lives. Father, please fortify us. Give us courage, strength and focus to continue pressing towards the mark of the high calling which is in you, Christ Jesus. Be with us throughout our day and allow us to feel your presence. We honor you for who you are in our lives.

In Jesus' name,

Amen

Reflection: How can you remain peaceful throughout your day?

The Holy Spirit Lives In Me

*Do you not know that you are the temple of God
and that the Spirit of God dwells in you?*
1 CORINTHIANS 3:16 (NLT)

Dear Gracious Heavenly Father,

I give you praise, honor and glory for your mercy and grace. Thank you for another day. Thank you for another opportunity to let my light shine from within. Father, I am certainly not perfect, however, when I fall, you are always right there. I know that you will never leave me nor forsake me. I have learned that I was not placed on this Earth to be alone. You created us to be in fellowship with one another because we are the body of Christ. In addition to being the body of Christ, I know that I am charged with taking care of my temple because that is where your Holy Spirit resides. Thank you for allowing me to feel your presence. Help me to be a beacon of light in the ways that would please you, Father. I am so grateful for your love and grace.

In Jesus' name,

Amen

Reflection: Reflect back to what you have eaten in the last 24 hours. What is one item that you are willing to give up in order to honor your temple? How will you replace those items to nourish yourself holistically?

DEVELOPING A PRAYER LIFE

Let Your Light Shine In Me

The light shines in the darkness, and the darkness can never extinguish it.
1 JOHN 1:5 (NLT)

Dear Gracious Heavenly Father,

This is the day that you have made, we shall rejoice and be glad in it. Father, we live in a world where darkness surrounds us, however, in your word you have taught us that the light shines in the darkness, and the darkness can never extinguish it.

We are that light. Help me to shine my light as a way to show that you reside in my heart and soul. Please fortify me so when dark times arise, I have the strength to push through and allow your light to shine through me and overcome the darkness. Thank you for being my light and guide. Help me to remain humble and teachable as I follow you along this journey. Please bless all those that I know and love across the globe. Please cover my family and friends today and allow us to continue to feel your presence in our lives.

In Jesus' name,

Amen

Reflection: What are some ways that you can show to others how God lives in your heart?

Purify My Spirit, God

> Have mercy on me, O God, because of your
> unfailing love. Because of your great compassion,
> blot out the stain of my sins. Wash me clean from
> my guilt. Purify me from my sin.
> PSALMS 51:1-2 (NLT)

Dear Gracious Heavenly Father,

Thank you for your mercy and grace. Father, I know I make mistakes and even sometimes I go against your will. I do not want to hurt your heart by doing things that I know are not good for me. Please forgive me, Father, for not listening and following your guidance. I realize that you love me unconditionally and your love is unfailing. Your compassion is beyond measure. Help me to honor my life by being obedient to you. Please cleanse me and make me whole again. I love you, Lord. Please bless every dear heart across the globe and their families. Help us all to be forgiving to others just as you have so graciously been to us time and time again.

In Jesus' name,

Amen

Reflection: How can you demonstrate obedience to God?

DEVELOPING A PRAYER LIFE

Spending Devoted Time With God

> But when you pray, go away by yourself, shut the door behind you, and pray to your Father in private. Then your Father, who sees everything, will reward you.
> MATTHEW 6:6 (NLT)

Dear Precious Heavenly Father,

Thank you for the gift of prayer. I am so grateful that I can come to you and share my worries and pain because you will be right there to comfort me. You desire is for me to cast all of my cares on you, so instead of carrying all of my burdens alone and on my own, I look to you. Father, I thank you for blessing me with a praying mother who taught us the importance of developing our own personal relationship and prayer life with you. Although you called her home to be with you, she left behind a strong spiritual legacy of faith, love, kindness, compassion and strength in you. I feel so blessed today and just want to say thank you. Thank you for all things.

In Jesus' name,

Amen

Reflection: Reflect on the life lessons that your parents/guardians have taught you. Describe the lesson that has had the biggest impact on you.

Help Me Meditate On You and Not My Mishaps

> Study this Book of Instruction continually. Meditate on it day and night so you will be sure to obey everything written in it. Only then will you prosper and succeed in all you do.
> JOSHUA 1:8 (NLT)

Dear Gracious Heavenly Father,

I give you praise, honor and glory for who you are in my life. Thank you for your word as it is a lamp unto my feet and a light unto my path. Father, you taught us to meditate on your word so that we can be closer to you and keep our focus on you, rather than our problems. Your desire is for us not to worry but yet worship you, rather than exalt the problem. When we focus on you, we fill our minds with positive thoughts and your ways. Thank you for reigning over my life. Thank you for direction and guidance. In you, I will continue to put my trust. I am grateful each day that you watch over and bless us as we learn and grow together. We give your name praise.

In Jesus' name,

Amen

Reflection: How do the scriptures help you navigate life's challenges?

DEVELOPING A PRAYER LIFE

Connecting With the Creator

> For ever since the world was created, people have seen the earth and sky. Through everything God made, they can clearly see his invisible qualities—his eternal power and divine nature.
> ROMANS 1:20 (NLT)

Dear Majestic Heavenly Father,

I stand in awe of you as you are mighty and worthy to be praised! In Romans 1:20, we are reminded of how we should connect the creation of our beautiful Earth with you, our creator. Your word tells us:

"For ever since the world was created, people have seen the earth and sky. Through everything God made, they can clearly see his invisible qualities—his eternal power and divine nature." So they have no excuse for not knowing God. Father, just yesterday as I was driving, I saw some of the most beautiful trees. The colors were so vivid that I had to slow down and acknowledge their beauty and your creation. The fall foliage, gorgeous clear, blue sky made me think about Psalms 24:1, *"The earth is the Lord's and everything in it. The world and all its people belong to you."* I am honored to be your child and belong to you. Thank you for showing up in ways all around me that are so evident and beautiful for me to experience each day of my life. I will continue to exalt your name and give you praise.

In Jesus' name,

Amen

Reflection: As you go out into nature, in what ways do you see examples of God's glory around you?

His Amazing Grace
(The Ultimate Sacrifice)

For God presented Jesus as the sacrifice for sin.
Romans 3:25 (NLT)

Dear Gracious Heavenly Father,

Thank you for your mercy and grace. I am so humbled to know that you made the ultimate sacrifice for my sins. In Romans 3:25, it explains to us that:

"For God presented Jesus as the sacrifice for sin." People are made right with God when they believe that Jesus sacrificed his life, shedding his blood. This sacrifice shows that God was being fair when he held back and did not punish those who sinned in times past, so therefore I am free indeed. I am forgiven through the shedding of the blood of Christ. I thank you for your amazing grace today because I can have a personal relationship with you that is all my own. Please help me to continue to follow you along this spiritual journey and celebrate the life that you have created for me. I will never cease to give you the praise, honor and glory due your name.

In Jesus' name,

Amen

Reflection: How will you honor the gift of your life to demonstrate that you are grateful for God's grace?

We Exalt You Jesus!

All nations will come to your light; mighty kings will come to see your radiance.
Isaiah 60:3 (NLT)

Dear Majestic Heavenly Father,

I worship you today and sing your praises because you are our true King! You are our Messiah! You reign over all nations. Your light pierces the darkness and creates a clear path for us to show others kindness, love and compassion. Help me, Father, to continue to be a beacon of light, love and hope for all those around me. Isaiah 60:3 tells us that:

"All nations will come to your light; mighty kings will come to see your radiance." As we walk along our journey with you, teach us to be a reflection of your light so that it is evident that surely goodness and mercy follows us. Your mercy is not something we need to chase. I am so grateful that your grace and mercy is given, if I simply seek you first. I give you thanks for all things and praise your name forever.

In Jesus' name,

Amen

Reflection: Take some time to reflect on the ways that you experience God. Take a picture and share it with your family and friends with hashtag:
#theearthisthelordsandthefullnessthereof

Let's Walk In God's Light Together

But if we walk in the light as He is in the light, we have fellowship with one another, and the blood of Jesus Christ His Son cleanses us from all sin.
1 JOHN 5:7

Dear Gracious Heavenly Father,

I come humbly before you today thanking you for all things. I want to thank you for your unconditional love when I fall short of your glory. Your word tells us:

"But if we are living in the light, as God is in the light, then we have fellowship with each other, and the blood of Jesus, his Son, cleanses us from all sin." Thank you for your forgiveness. You are so merciful. Please help me, Father, to let my light shine and live a life that honors you.

In Jesus' name,

Amen

Reflection: Thank God for his love and forgiveness. We have the opportunity to make positive changes in our lives every day. Describe the small change that you would like to ask God to help you make today to start anew.

Prayers of Comfort

All Things Are Possible With Christ

"I can do all things through Christ which strengthens me."
PHILIPPIANS 4:13 (KJV)

Dear Gracious Heavenly Father,

You are so mighty and so awesome! I am in awe of your grace. Father, in Philippians 4:13, your word encourages us by saying, "I can do all things through Christ which strengthens me." I specifically remember when you called my earthly father home. His transition to heaven took place on October 19, 2011, which inevitably meant that his celebration of life services would take place shortly thereafter. Our family held the services on my birthday, October 25, 2011. I remember everyone being concerned about my well-being and how difficult it may have been for me. I told my sisters, "If this is what needs to be done, I will gladly honor Daddy in this way." Father, I distinctly remember, when October 25, 2011 arrived, you gave me so much strength, power and courage to face the day. Although my heart was heavy that my earthly father was no longer here with us physically, I was comforted by your unconditional love, the love of my family and village. You gave me peace on that day that surpassed all understanding and I now know that I can do all things through Christ that strengthens me. Please comfort those who may have heavy hearts today. Allow them to feel your presence. Thank you for always being at the center of my life. I bless your name forever.

In Jesus' name,

Amen

Reflection: My earthly father was a generous man who loved his family and therefore, I honor both his legacy and my spiritual walk with Christ by serving others in need. How will you honor your ancestors?

God's Unfailing Love

Each morning I will sing with joy about your unfailing love. For you have been my refuge, a place of safety when I am in distress.
PSALMS 59:16 (NLT)

Dear Precious Heavenly Father,

You are my refuge and strength. In times of trouble, you will protect me. In Psalm 59:16, I learned:

"For you have been my refuge, a place of safety when I am in distress." I am so grateful for your unfailing love especially in times of trouble. Father, thank you for being my comforter. I will sing praises to you for your loving kindness and the faithfulness that you consistently show to me. Your power is infinite and you are so mighty. Father, because you are omniscient, you already know all about the storms that I will face, so therefore, please fortify and strengthen me so that my life is a reflection of your power and strength as I endure. Help me to never cease to give you the praise, honor and glory due your name.

In Jesus' name,

Amen

Reflection: Listen to soothing music that speaks to and comforts your soul.

God Heals Broken Hearts

*He heals the brokenhearted and
binds up their wounds.*
PSALMS 147:3 (NLT)

Dear Gracious Heavenly Father,

You are our healer. You are our source and strength. You see all that we go through each day. Thank you for your unconditional love because there is no comparison of your love for us. When we are brokenhearted, thank you for offering us a place of refuge from the pain. I am so grateful that your embrace provides comfort and healing for our wounded souls. Please restore us, Father, and even those who may be feeling lonely today. Help them to know that you are right by their side. You are our Jehovah Rapha, our healer, and you will make our hearts whole again. I declare restoration for all those in the Angel Network, my family and friends. Heal the weary in heart and spirit, Father. Fall afresh on us. We love you today for your mercy and grace.

In Jesus' name,

Amen

Reflection: Draw a heart on a piece of paper. Write the names of each family member that you would like to remember in a loving way. Reflect on the ways that they have touched your life and allow God to comfort you in the moment. Hang the heart wherever you would like in your home.

PRAYER OF COMFORT

Replenish Our Souls

For I have satiated the weary soul, and I have replenished every sorrowful soul."
JEREMIAH 31:25 (KJV)

Dear Gracious Heavenly Father,

Thank you, Jesus, for this beautiful day! This is a day filled with brand new mercies just for me. Father, you are our comforter, refuge and strength. I thank you for being there for me when I am weary and feeling overwhelmed. In Jeremiah 31:25, you teach us that you will refresh the weary and satisfy the faint. I am encouraged to know that in you there is restoration and unexpected blessings waiting for me. Help me to just rest and abide in you. Thank you for your presence in our lives. Father, please continue to watch over and bless my family and friends. We love you wholeheartedly.

In Jesus' name,

Amen

Reflection: It's rejuvenation day! What can you do for yourself to replenish your soul today?

God Is Our Refuge

The Lord is good, a strong refuge when trouble comes. He is close to those who trust in him.
NAHUM 1:7 (NLT)

Dear Gracious Heavenly Father,

I am so grateful for your mercy and grace. You are so merciful to us. When I am overwhelmed, I look to you because I know you are my refuge and strength. You provide me with such comfort. Thank you for reminding me that when I am weak, you are strong. Thank you for teaching me to trust you even when the situation is full of uncertainty. Please continue to watch over and bless my family as we go throughout our day. Help us to show love to one another as you have shown us. We honor you and glorify your name.

In Jesus' name,

Amen

Reflection: **What are some ways to show love to the individuals in your life and honor God?**

Honoring Mom: Our Queen Warrior

Nuggets of Wisdom

Blessed are they that mourn: for they shall be comforted.
MATTHEW 5:4 (KJV)

Dear Precious Heavenly Father,

Thank you for this beautiful day! I thank you for your protection and love. Lord, I thank you for all the things that I have that you have given me the strength and fortitude to obtain. God, at this time my heart is heavy because I miss my parents immensely, particularly my mother. She was your faithful servant. God, you said, blessed are they that mourn and the memory of the just is blessed. Lord, thank you for blessing my siblings and me with a saved mother, a prayer warrior, a virtuous woman of God and a faithful wife who was dedicated to her family. Lord, she taught us the gift of prayer through devotion. She ensured that our lives would be anchored in you. I remain grateful today for the lessons she taught us about you, Lord. So, Father, as I begin my day, please help me to lean on you for comfort, guidance and know that you will give not only me, but all those in need, peace that surpasses all understanding. My faith has not wavered in your powerful ability to heal because I believe in your promises. I love you, Lord.

In Jesus' name,

Amen

> *Reflection: If you could write a letter to a loved one in heaven, what would you say? Take some time out today to reflect on your thoughts and write your letter to them.*

Life Lessons From Mom

Every good gift and every perfect gift is from above, and comes down from the Father of lights, with whom there is no variation or shadow of turning.
JAMES 1:17 (NLT)

Dear Precious Heavenly Father,

Thank you for every good and perfect gift from above. Thank you for blessing my sisters and brother and me with a saved mother who realized the gift of prayer. Our mother realized that knowing you and acknowledging who you are in our lives helps us to maintain a blessed life. Thank you for never changing and for sending your light down from heaven onto us. Help us to look at our lives and think on whatsoever things are lovely and pure and maintain an attitude of gratitude for all that you have given us. Thank you for being our provider. Let us not take things for granted but to always be thankful. Bless us this day. Please keep us safe from harm. You are our King!

In Jesus' name,

Amen

Reflection: Draw/Paint a picture that expresses how you honor Christ in your life.

Memories of Mom

I just wanted to take a moment to share a short personal story with you about my mother. When my siblings and I were younger, my mother taught us a grace for dinner and a special one for dessert. For those of you who aren't aware, my mother received her crown and is resting in God's arms. Her "angel-versary" was May 24, 2018. As you can imagine, I miss her immensely. Whenever we had ice cream or some of her delicious homemade pound cake, she would always have us pray: Every good gift is from above. In Jesus' name, Amen.

Do you know that I discovered through my devotional time, that my mother taught us that precious grace directly from the scripture in James 1:17? She was such a virtuous woman of God. We were so blessed to have been raised with love and guidance to know the Lord. I'm sharing this story with you because the scripture was a part of my special devotion and it just brought back such sweet memories. So, God, thank you for giving us Mommy for as long as we had her and help us to continue to be grateful for every good gift from above.

In Jesus' name,

Amen

I Would Also Like To Share A Personal Story About My Father, Ronald M. Ingram, Sr.

In listening to Dr. Tony Evans, a powerful spiritual leader who has blessed my spiritual journey through his coherent teaching and preaching, I was very touched by what he said in his timely message regarding our heavenly father and all of us who were blessed to have an earthly father. I shared with my sisters that we were so blessed because our father did cover us in times of crisis. I specifically remember when a contractor ruined things at my home and I went to my dad. He did not hesitate to help. I remember asking him to pray with me and he got on his knees. Growing up, we didn't have to worry about whether we were going to eat, have running water or whether the lights would be kept on....we were always cared for and loved. In Matthew 6:34, Dr. Tony Evans reminded us to not worry about tomorrow. How many times do we say this to one another even now, when we have trials or tribulations that come up in our lives? My sisters and I say to each other: Mommy would say.... "Don't borrow any worry from tomorrow." So much of what Mommy taught us was direct teaching from the scriptures and the Word of God. How richly blessed are we to have had both a strong father who was a protector, a provider and supporter and a saved mother who instilled in us the importance of developing a personal relationship with our heavenly father?!

Although we miss our parents immensely, we carry them in our hearts today with all that they have taught us. My prayer today is that you are comforted by the nuggets of wisdom and spiritual foundation that was created for you by those who were blessed with parents, loving caregivers and trailblazers who have touched your life. Remember what they poured into you and pass it on to uplift the next generation.

ROBIN K. INGRAM

Don't Borrow Any Worry From Tomorrow

Therefore do not worry about tomorrow, for tomorrow will worry about its own things. Sufficient for the day is its own trouble.
Matthew 6:34 (NIV)

Dear Gracious Heavenly Father,

I come before you with a grateful heart. I thank you for all things. I am especially grateful for being raised by a prayer warrior who was your faithful servant and she spent time studying your Word so that she could teach my siblings and me. Today's scripture is from Matthew 6:34 and our mother used to say to us: "Don't borrow any worry from tomorrow." Her guidance was taken directly from the Word of God like so many other life lessons that we have been taught. I give you glory, honor and praise today, Father, because although my mother is in heaven, she leaves behind a strong legacy of excellence for us to follow that is grounded in your Word. So today, I take a moment to just honor my mother's dedicated role as our anointed teacher and also a faithful servant of God. We bless your name forever more.

In Jesus' name,

Amen

Reflection: If you find yourself worrying today, remember the words of my mother, which were based on Matthew 6:34 and remind yourself: "We will not borrow any worry from tomorrow." Practice being mindful by staying present in the moment.

Expressing Gratitude & Love Through Prayer

ROBIN K. INGRAM

My Life Is In Your Hands

"For I know the plans I have for you, plans to prosper you and not to harm you, plans to give you hope and a future."
JEREMIAH 29:11 (NIV)

Dear Gracious Heavenly Father,

O Lord, I will honor and praise your name, for you are my God. You do such wonderful things! You planned them long ago, and now you have accomplished them. You knew me because you created me in my mother's womb. You crafted each gift and talent that I possess. Help me, Father, to use those gifts to glorify you and draw closer to you as I serve others. Thank you for your word in Jeremiah 29:11, where you tell us:

"For I know the plans I have for you, plans to prosper you and not to harm you, plans to give you hope and a future." What good would it profit us to gain this whole world but lose our souls? Thank you for protecting our hearts, minds and souls, Father. Thank you for giving us hope to persevere despite all that goes on around us. Help us to remember that where your spirit dwells, there is peace, freedom and love. Let us rest and abide in you today and always.

In Jesus' name,

Amen

Reflection: Arise with a grateful heart and end your day by being thankful for all of your blessings.

EXPRESSING GRATITUDE & LOVE THROUGH PRAYER

Grateful For Forgiveness

You forgave the guilt of your people— yes, you covered all their sins.
PSALMS 85:2 (NLT)

Dear Gracious Heavenly Father,

Today I come humbly before you with an earnest heart thanking you for your forgiveness. So much is happening in the world around us. There is tragedy and illness. These stressors can cause our anxiety to heighten and we sometimes want to take matters into our own hands. Thank you, God, for covering my sins when I step out of your will, even when I have heard your voice guiding me but I am still disobedient to your leading. Thank you for giving me another chance to worship you in all truth. Yesterday is gone, however today, we can start anew and move forward with you by our side. We honor you today, Messiah. Please bless all those who desire to remain in your will. Strengthen us in you.

In Jesus' name,

Amen

Reflection: Our God is forgiving. Who would you like to ask for forgiveness in your life so you are able to start anew? Remember to forgive yourself first.

ROBIN K. INGRAM

Grateful To Experience God's Greatness

For as the waters fill the sea, the earth will be filled with an awareness of your glory.
HABAKKUK 2:14 (NLT)

Dear Gracious Heavenly Father,

I give you praise and honor for this glorious day! As I arise and I am greeted by the beautiful sunshine that you have allowed me to see, I am grateful for its warmth and beauty. Knowing you is not just about learning and memorizing scriptures. Having a personal relationship with you, making room for you in our lives creates the opportunity to experience you authentically. What a truly divine gift! Habakkuk 2:14 tells us:

"For as the waters fill the sea, the earth will be filled with an awareness of your glory" so therefore everyone, everywhere will know and experience your greatness. I stand in awe of you even today as I look around at the beautiful trees and leaves and vivid colors. You are our Creator. You are our Alpha and Omega. We worship you forever.

In Jesus' name,

Amen

---

*Reflection: **Take time today to make connections with the creativity in nature gifted to us by our Creator.***

EXPRESSING GRATITUDE & LOVE THROUGH PRAYER

Empathy vs. Sympathy

Carry each other's burdens, and in this way you will fulfill the law of Christ.
GALATIANS 6:2 (NIV)

Dear Precious Heavenly Father,

I come before you today with a grateful heart. I thank you for always being there for me. Father, you allow me to be cast my cares on you because you care for me. Your word, in Galatians 6:2, reads:

"Carry each other's burdens, and in this way you will fulfill the law of Christ." I thank you for increasing my faith and ability to empathize with others when they are experiencing difficulties in their lives. I am also grateful for being able to know the difference between empathy and sympathy. Help us, Father, to be authentic advocates of compassion. Please enhance our ability to empathize with others and make true connections in challenging times, especially times of sorrow. Create pure hearts in each of us to truly be willing to stand with our brother and sister by turning love into an action. Thank you for your purposeful instruction for our lives, Father. We love you and honor your presence each day.

In Jesus' name,

Amen

Reflection: How can knowing the difference between empathy and sympathy enhance your relationships?

Grateful For My Blessings

Don't store up treasures here on earth, where moths eat them and rust destroys them, and where thieves break in and steal.
MATTHEW 6:19 (NLT)

Dear Precious Heavenly Father,

Thank you for all things. Thank you for every blessing that you have given me. Father, it can be so easy to get distracted by worldly possessions and desire to acquire many different things. In Matthew 6:19, your word teaches us:

"Don't store up treasures here on earth, where moths eat them and rust destroys them, and where thieves break in and steal." Help me to remember that only what I do for you will last. In you, there is no lack because you will supply all of my needs. I can live with the assurance of knowing that I am covered by your protection and love; therefore, I can prioritize my focus on the building of your kingdom, while still remaining a beneficiary of your provision. I will forever be grateful for your grace.

In Jesus' name,

Amen

Reflection:
In your journal, title a page "blessings." Make a list of all of God's blessings given to you and your family. Hang the list in your prayer closet. Use it to practice gratitude.

EXPRESSING GRATITUDE & LOVE THROUGH PRAYER

God, Thank You For Being There For Me

But it is no shame to suffer for being a Christian. Praise God for the privilege of being called by his name!
1 PETER 4:16 (NLT)

Dear Gracious Heavenly Father,

I give you praise, honor and glory for who you are in my life. Thank you for making the ultimate sacrifice so that I may have eternal life. When I was a little girl, I wrote a song entitled: "I'm not ashamed of the Gospel of Jesus Christ." Thank you for placing that song in my spirit because it still is true today. Although we may have times when we suffer or are hurting, you want us to know as you said in your word: "But it is no shame to suffer for being a Christian. Praise God for the privilege of being called by his name!" Sometimes when we suffer or experience tribulations, it gives us an opportunity to get even closer to you, Father, and we can just wait for you to show up in our lives. We do not suffer in vain, for out of our pain comes powerful strength. Thank you for fortifying us, protecting us and teaching us how to glorify you. Thank you for your many blessings. We magnify your name forever.

In Jesus' name,

Amen

Reflection: If you could encourage a fellow Christian today who is experiencing a challenging situation, how would you help them?

Click this link to access my video entitled:
Attitude of Gratitude https://youtu.be/wPJzi2mJRBM

Agape Love

"A new commandment I give unto you, That ye love one another; as I have loved you, that ye also love one another."
JOHN 13:34 (NIV)

Dear Gracious Heavenly Father,

You have shown me through your sacrifice and unconditional love how to demonstrate that love to others. It is an action. Thank you for being such an awesome example so that I would know how to treat others. I ask, Father, that you strengthen me when I need to love those who have mistreated me because I know that is the real challenge. You are not impressed by what I know, you are watching what I do. Please let my deeds be demonstrations of your love in my life. Please continue to be ever present in my life so that I may show love and uplift others. I thank you for my family, friends and Angel Network. I am so blessed and do not take it for granted. You are a merciful God and we praise your name.

In Jesus' name,

Amen

Reflection: How can you express God's love to others?

EXPRESSING GRATITUDE & LOVE THROUGH PRAYER

Show Kindness and Love

If I could speak all the languages of earth and of angels, but didn't love others, I would only be a noisy gong or a clanging cymbal.
1 CORINTHIANS 13:1 (NLT)

Dear Gracious Heavenly Father,

Thank you for the gift of your love. I have learned through your word that two of the most important commandments are for me to love you and others. You have shown me how it feels to be loved unconditionally because even when I am disobedient to your word, you are still there for me. Father, you have given each one of us special and unique gifts. Your desire is for me to use those gifts in a loving way. Help me, Father, to demonstrate your love as I go throughout my day. God, you have taught me in your word, in 1 Corinthians 13:1:

"If I could speak all the languages of earth and of angels, but didn't love others, I would only be a noisy gong or a clanging cymbal." Instead of showing up in the world as unnecessary noise, help me, Father, to show kindness and love that comforts others. Please continue to bless and watch over all those that I know and love. Protect and cover them today.

In Jesus' name,

Amen

Reflection: Describe your God-given gifts. How do you use them?

Representing God's Love

Do what is right, to love mercy, and to walk humbly with your God.
MICAH 6:8 (NLT)

Dear Heavenly Father,

I come before you today with a spirit of humility. I desire to live a life that honors you. Father, please help me put Micah 6:8b into practice in an authentic way. Your word says:

"O people, the Lord has told you what is good, and this is what he requires of you: to do what is right, to love mercy, and to walk humbly with your God." Father, I desire to do what is right and just in your sight. Help me to also walk humbly with you each day so that it is evident that you live in my heart and soul. When I show up in the world, my spirit and the way I treat others should be a representation of your love.

Lord, please continue to bless us all as we go out into the world. Help us to love one another as you love us. We will continue to bless your name forever.

In Jesus' name,

Amen

Reflection: What is unconditional love?

EXPRESSING GRATITUDE & LOVE THROUGH PRAYER

Grateful For God's Presence In My Life

Surely goodness and mercy shall follow me all the days of my life: and I will dwell in the house of the Lord forever.
PSALMS 23:6 (KJV)

Dear Precious Heavenly Father,

I give you praise, honor and glory today, for you are our Shepherd. Not only do you protect us each day, but you also love us unconditionally. As human beings, we tend to cause hurt whether it is intentional or unintentional, however, your love for us is forever. You will never leave us. We can have confidence in knowing that if we put our faith and trust in you, our future is certain because it is in your hands. In Psalms 23:6, we learn about how you will be with us forever. In your word it tells us that:

"Surely goodness and mercy shall follow me all the days of my life: and I will dwell in the house of the Lord forever." I am so grateful that I can feel your presence in my life because it is such a comfort. It gives me such peace. Father, please continue to watch over and bless all those that I know and love. We honor you today and always.

In Jesus' name,

Amen

Reflection: How has God shown up for you when you exercised your faith in him?

Peace That Surpasses All Understanding

For the mountains shall depart and the hills be removed, but My kindness shall not depart from you, nor shall my covenant of peace be removed," says the Lord, who has mercy on you.
Isaiah 54:10 (NLT)

Dear Gracious Heavenly Father,

I come before you today with a grateful heart. Thank you for your unconditional love for me. Thank you for your faithfulness and willingness to be a force that is steadfast in my life. When everything else around me seems to be chaotic, I thank you for creating a sense of calm. You are my refuge and strength. You give me peace that surpasses all understanding. Help me to remember to trust you with all my heart and just rest in you. We honor you today for continuing to watch over and bless our families and friends. We magnify your name.

In Jesus' name,

Amen

Reflection: It is random acts of kindness day! Randomly choose 3 people in your life that you want to show kindness to today and decide how you will be a blessing to them.

EXPRESSING GRATITUDE & LOVE THROUGH PRAYER

Loving Traits of a Christian

Therefore, as the elect of God, holy and beloved, put on tender mercies, kindness, humility, meekness, longsuffering.
COLOSSIANS 3:12 (NIV)

Dear Gracious Heavenly Father,

Thank you for your mercy and grace. Compassion, kindness, gentleness and humility are all traits that a Christian has as we grow closer to you spiritually. In your word, Father, you teach us that the way we treat others is a reflection of our love and commitment to you. Help us to "show up" in the world in our relationships and interactions with others in ways that reflect the unconditional love that you have for us. Thank you for being so merciful and for showing us the path that you have chosen for us. We honor you as our Messiah.

In Jesus' name,

Amen

Reflection: How will it be evident to others that God lives in your heart?

Cautiously Use the Power of Your Words

*A soft answer turns away wrath,
But a harsh word stirs up anger.*
PROVERBS 15:1 (NIV)

Dear Precious Heavenly Father,

Today is the day that you have made, let us rejoice and be glad in it. I give you praise, honor and glory for another beautiful day and the opportunity to praise your glorious name. In Proverbs, you teach us that there is power in our words so therefore it is so important to use wisdom and respond cautiously with you as our guide. As you have taught us, a soft answer will turn away wrath. Help us, Father, to let the words of our mouth and the meditation of our hearts be acceptable in thy sight. Fortify us to maintain a calm confidence even in the face of adversity. You are our rock and strong tower. Thank you for allowing us to lean on you. Please bless every individual who is a part of our Angel Network, my family and friends. We bless your majestic name today and give you praise.

In Jesus' name,

Amen

Reflection: It is not always easy to maintain a calm confidence. Today, practice staying connected with Christ and think on positive things when situations become challenging by implementing my P.T.R.L. strategy: Pray, Think and then Respond with Love.

EXPRESSING GRATITUDE & LOVE THROUGH PRAYER

Be a Testament of God's Love

For there is one God and one Mediator between God and men, the Man Christ Jesus.
1 TIMOTHY 2:5 (NIV)

Dear Gracious Heavenly Father,

You are our SOURCE. I give you praise, honor and glory today and have a heart full of gratitude for you making the ultimate sacrifice to give your life so that I may be free. I am so grateful. As I go throughout my day, please help me to show my gratitude by living as a testament of your love by sharing with others all about you as I pray for their well being. Father, you have plans for us and want the very best for our lives. Help us to stay divinely connected to you so that you may order our steps. Thank you for your unconditional love for us. Please bless every precious soul that is impacted by the outreach. We worship you today for you are worthy to be praised.

In Jesus' name,

Amen

Reflection: God has blessed each one of us with special gifts. What are your special gifts and talents? How do you use them in your community?

Demonstrate Love Everywhere You Go

Seek the Lord, all you meek of the earth, who have upheld His justice. Seek righteousness, seek humility.
ZEPHANIAH 2:3 (NIV)

Dear Gracious Heavenly Father,

Thank you for your mercy and grace. Thank you for all that you have given me and how you continue to bless me each day. Father, with the love that you show us, it is your desire that we live our lives humbly and demonstrate love to one another. Love is an action word. Thank you for showing up for me, for my family and for being our rock. I remain grateful. As we go into the days ahead, I pray a prayer of protection over all those that I know and love. Encamp your angels all around us and please place a hedge of protection around our homes and everywhere we go, Father. Let us continue to look to you and listen for your voice.

In Jesus' name,

Amen

Reflection: Walk through your home and pray for God's protection over your family.

EXPRESSING GRATITUDE & LOVE THROUGH PRAYER

Unconditional Love

Be on your guard; stand firm in the faith; be courageous; be strong.
1 CORINTHIANS 16:13 (NIV)

Dear Gracious Heavenly Father,

Thank you for being my hope. With you by my side, there is no reason to fear. Standing on your word is an exercise in being courageous and showing my faith in you, Father. I realize that distractions may arise and take my focus away from you, however, I ask, Father, that you strengthen me and please help me to have unshakable faith because you are my source. In you, I put my trust. Help me to guard my heart and mind so that I may do everything with love as you have taught us in 1 Corinthians 16:13. Thank you for your unconditional love for us and new mercies each day. Please bless every dear heart that I know and love. Cover them. I honor you today and always.

In Jesus' name,

Amen

Reflection: How can you demonstrate God's love in your daily life in an actionable way?

Our Compassionate God

> Because of the Lord's great love we are not consumed, for his compassions never fail. They are new every morning; great is your faithfulness.
> LAMENTATIONS 3:22-23 (NIV)

Dear Gracious Heavenly Father,

Thank you for your love and faithfulness. You give us brand new mercies each day and I am so grateful. In your word, in Lamentations 3:22-23, you taught us:

"Because of the Lord's great love we are not consumed, for his compassions never fail. They are new every morning; great is your faithfulness." "The Lord is my portion," says my soul, "Therefore I hope in Him!" Help us to be encouraged, remain hopeful and maintain an attitude of gratitude for each blessing each day. We give you all the praise, honor and glory due your name.

In Jesus' name,

Amen

Reflection: Complete this statement. Today, I am grateful for_____.

Servitude, Leadership & Wisdom

ROBIN K. INGRAM

Living a Purpose-Filled Life

"Therefore, go and make disciples of all the nations, baptizing them in the name of the Father and the Son and the Holy Spirit.
MATTHEW 28:19 (NLT)

Dear Heavenly Father,

Thank you for your guidance. Thank you for giving us a purpose-filled life. Along this journey, we are expected to touch the lives of others through you. In Matthew 28:19, you tell us:

"Therefore, go and make disciples of all the nations, baptizing them in the name of the Father and the Son and the Holy Spirit." You are our King and therefore each Christian is called according to your purpose to be a missionary to make disciples. Our charge is meaningful and it reaches across nations. It is a part of your grand design because you are our Messiah.

Spreading the gospel and faith is our mission and we thank you, Father, for the opportunity to uplift the lives of others and give your name praise, honor and glory.

In Jesus' name,

Amen

Reflection: How would you describe your spiritual mission?

SERVITUDE, LEADERSHIP & WISDOM

Share the Good News

Work hard so you can present yourself to God and receive his approval. Be a good worker, one who does not need to be ashamed and who correctly explains the word of truth.
2 TIMOTHY 2:15 (NLT)

Dear Gracious Heavenly Father,

It is such an honor and blessing to know you. Thank you for this beautiful day and for another opportunity to represent you in the work that I do as I strive for excellence. In your word you explain to us:

"Work hard so you can present yourself to God and receive his approval. Be a good worker, one who does not need to be ashamed and who correctly explains the word of truth." I have learned, Father, we must first be a student of the word and study it, before we can become the teacher. When we understand your word, we are able to apply it in circumstances of spiritual warfare. We are better prepared because we step into battle with our swords, (the Bible), raised high to defeat the attack of the enemy. Help us to meet your approval as we stay in the faith and invite more people to get to know you as you remain at the center of our lives. We bless your magnificent name today and always.

In Jesus' name,

Amen

Reflection: Which scripture speaks to your testimony? How has studying the Word of God enhanced your life?

I Am God's Spirit-Filled Vessel

So whether you eat or drink or whatever you do, do it all for the glory of God.
1 CORINTHIANS 10:31 (NLT)

Dear Gracious Heavenly Father,

I give you praise, honor and glory. Thank you for choosing me with all of my flaws and imperfections because in your eyes, I am a masterpiece. I am your masterpiece, here to glorify you and be used as your vessel in whatever I do. In your word, in 1 Corinthians 10:31, you tell us that:

"So whether you eat or drink or whatever you do, do it all for the glory of God." So, Father, please help me to remember that my life is a gift from you. Help me to honor my life in a purposeful way as I maintain my faith in you for all things. Please remember all those who are struggling in silence today. Comfort and restore the hearts and minds of your people. Please expand the Angel Network across the globe and allow us to represent you in beautiful ways. Cover my family and friends with your precious blood.

In Jesus' name,

Amen

Reflection: Stand in front of a mirror and tell yourself: I am a masterpiece made by God. Write this statement on a post-it and place it in the mirror as a daily affirmation.

SERVITUDE, LEADERSHIP & WISDOM

Serve With Honor, Warrior

*Then, calling the crowd to join his disciples,
he said, "If any of you wants to be my follower,
you must give up your own way,
take up your cross, and follow me.*
MARK 8:34 (NLT)

Dear Heavenly Father,

In your word, in Mark 8:34, you speak to us about surrendering our lives and following you. Your word also says:

"If you try to hang on to your life, you will lose it. But if you give up your life for my sake and for the sake of the Good News, you will save it." (Matthew 16:25) So many times I have taken my concerns into my own hands without realizing that true surrender is giving my life to you, sharing about the gospel and allowing you to guide and protect me. You are my Jehovah Jireh, my provider, therefore in you, there is no lack, I will have everything that I need. You are my Jehovah Rapha, therefore by your stripes, I am healed. Please fortify me holistically, Father, so that I may be a strong warrior who follows you so that I may live with you forever in eternity. I will never cease to give you all the praise due your name.

In Jesus' name,

Amen

Reflection: Are there any organizations in your community that you would like to serve? How can you allow God's light shine through you as you serve?

ROBIN K. INGRAM

Be a Wise Leader

The fear of the Lord is the beginning of wisdom and the knowledge of the holy is understanding.
PROVERBS 9:10 (NIV)

Dear Gracious Heavenly Father,

You are our loving Father. You desire for us to have the best in this life. As we travel along life's journey, there will be many different decisions to make. The decisions we make can often have a major impact on our ability to be fruitful, successful and live a full life. Proverbs 9:10 tells us:

"The fear of the Lord is the beginning of wisdom and the knowledge of the holy is understanding." Father, you do not want us to fear you in an unhealthy way, but you want us to look to you for guidance and direction. Help us, Father, to be wise enough to follow in the righteous path that you have created for our lives. Knowing you will help us to gain insight, knowledge and understand what it truly means to be wise. Thank you for being our anchor.

In Jesus' name,

Amen

Reflection: How will you include God in the decisions that you make for your life?

SERVITUDE, LEADERSHIP & WISDOM

God Gives Us the Wisdom to Lead

"Remain in me, and I will remain in you. For a branch cannot produce fruit if it is severed from the vine, and you cannot be fruitful unless you remain in me."
JOHN 15:4 (NIV)

Dear Precious Heavenly Father,

You are our awesome King! You reign over our lives with patience and love. As my spiritual growth is shaped by the application of your word in my life, please help me to understand that you desire for us to bear quality fruit from the branches of our trees and not be concerned about the quantity. As John 15:4 tells us:

"Remain in me, and I will remain in you. For a branch cannot produce fruit if it is severed from the vine, and you cannot be fruitful unless you remain in me." Give us the wisdom to abide in you, learn of your ways so that we may bring others to truly know you. Help us to share your gospel and not be concerned with how many "likes or followers" we have on our social media but rather, focus on who has come to know you as a result of responding to the calling on our lives. Let us see that abiding in you as we seek to fulfill our purpose in you, will truly define success. Please bless our families, friends and all those who desire to experience you on a personal level. Thank you for your constant presence in my life. It brings me such peace. I love you, Lord, and give you praise.

In Jesus' name,

Amen

Reflection: Try not to allow technology to rule your life by limiting your exposure to social media each day.

God Is Our Anchor

If you are wise and understand God's ways, prove it by living an honorable life doing good works with humility that comes from wisdom.
JAMES 3:13 (NLT)

Dear Gracious Heavenly Father,

Thank you for your mercy and grace. I give you praise, honor and glory for you are our true King! You are so worthy to be praised. Father, I thank you for the opportunity to attend higher institutions of learning and use those learning experiences to shape my life today. However, Lord, help me to realize that true wisdom is finding the good in others and maintaining a spirit of humility as I fulfill my life's purpose. You are my anchor. Help me to look to you consistently for guidance and direction. I place my life in your hands and pray that you bless, anoint and expand that which you have assigned to me as part of my life's purpose. Strengthen me to serve with a spirit of humility and grace. I sing praises to you today and forever more.

In Jesus' name,

Amen

Reflection: Think about this quote, from Chadwick Boseman,

"Purpose is an essential element of you. It is the reason you are on the planet at this particular time in history. Your very existence is wrapped up in the things you are here to fulfill." How will you serve others today?

SERVITUDE, LEADERSHIP & WISDOM

Remain Teachable

*Be not wise in thine own eyes:
fear the Lord and depart from evil.*
PROVERBS 3:7 (KJV)

Dear Gracious Heavenly Father,

How blessed are we to know you and to be loved by you? I give you praise, honor and glory today, for you are our guide. Father, thank you for being my foundation. Thank you for allowing me to hear your voice. Help me to continue to push my own pride aside and look to you for wisdom, because in your word you tell us:

"Be not wise in thine own eyes: fear the Lord and depart from evil." It is your desire for us to acknowledge you in all of our ways and you will direct our path. I am so grateful to know that I am not on this journey alone. Help me Father, to remain teachable and have a positive impact on those around me. I thank you for being your vessel to serve your people. Father, please bring peace and comfort to our families and to this world. We believe in your word and stand on your promises. We love you Lord.

In Jesus' name,

Amen

Reflection: As we lean on God to lead us along our journey, what are some actions that we can take in order to remain teachable?

Success Defined Through the Eyes of God

"So humble yourselves under the mighty power of God, and at the right time he will lift you up in honor."
1 PETER 5:6 (NLT)

Dear Gracious Heavenly Father,

I come humbly before you today with a pure heart and a new found understanding about success, humility and how we are seen in this world through your eyes. Father, I thank you for your infinite wisdom. Thank you for teaching me to have a calm confidence in you that is neither haughty or insecure. Allow me to truly apply 1 Peter 5:6 to my life as it says:

"So humble yourselves under the mighty power of God, and at the right time he will lift you up in honor." Please allow me to define success (through your eyes) by fulfilling my God-given purpose of what you have called me to do with a spirit of humility. Give me patience to follow your lead until you ordain my elevation in you. Where you lead, I will follow. Thank you for reigning over my life. Thank you for keeping me safe and providing guidance for my journey. I bless your name today and forever more.

In Jesus' name,

Amen

Reflection: How do you define success as a child of God?

The Body of Christ; Serving Others

So that there should be no division in the body, but that its parts should have equal concern for each other. If one part suffers, every part suffers with it; if one part is honored, every part rejoices with it. Now you are the body of Christ, and each one of you is a part of it.
1 Corinthians 12: 25-27 (NIV)

Dear Gracious Heavenly Father,

Thank you for this beautiful day. I come humbly before you thanking you for the gifts that you have given me. In your word, you teach us that we are to be unified as one body in Christ and use our gifts to uplift, encourage and help others with a spirit of humility as we glorify you. Help me, Jesus, to use the gifts that you gave me to serve in a spirit of love. In the days ahead, please continue to give us the guidance that we need in order to best serve you as we serve others. As we acknowledge you in all of our ways, please strengthen us and give us the wisdom to be wise in making sound decisions along our path. Thank you for being our hope, protection and Messiah. We love you. Please remember every dear heart that is touched across the globe by the Angel Network, my family and friends. We will always give you the praise, honor and glory due your name.

In Jesus' name,

Amen

Reflection: Do you have a serving heart? Ask God to bless your gifts to be anointed in service to the building of his kingdom.

Renewing the Mind

"And be not conformed to this world: but be ye transformed by the renewing of your mind, that ye may prove what is that good, and acceptable, and perfect, will of God."
Romans 12:2 (KJV)

Dear Gracious Heavenly Father,

Thank you for being my guide. Thank you for creating me to think and have a spirit of discernment in order to make wise decisions about my life. I thank you for the patience and love that you have shown me as I diligently work on renewing my mind by keeping it focused on you. Father, thank you for your word in Romans 12:2 where it reads:

"And be not conformed to this world: but be ye transformed by the renewing of your mind, that ye may prove what is that good, and acceptable, and perfect, will of God." You have shown me the importance of maintaining a calm confidence in you, so that when situations arise, I am able to respond rather than just react. Thank you for your wisdom and for filling me with a desire to maintain a healthy balance in my life. I pray for all those who need a renewing of the mind today. I ask, Father, that you fall afresh on them. Allow them to feel your presence in their lives. I ask these things and give you praise.

In Jesus' name,

Amen

Reflection: Through God's gentle guidance, ask for renewal of your mind and remain trusting of his plan for your life.

SERVITUDE, LEADERSHIP & WISDOM

Foundation of True Knowledge

*Fear of the Lord is the foundation of true knowledge,
but fools despise wisdom and discipline.*
PROVERBS 1:7 (NLT)

Dear Gracious Heavenly Father,

I stand in awe of you, your wisdom, unfailing grace, and mercy. Father, I am so grateful for your unconditional love for us and how you made the ultimate sacrifice so that I might be free. When I was growing up, I was not "afraid" of my parents but rather, I had a respectful fear because I knew that there were consequences for my behavior. I also knew that my parents were much wiser than me; they were prepared to teach me so much more about life than I could ever imagine. Proverbs 1:7 says:

"Fear of the Lord is the foundation of true knowledge, but fools despise wisdom and discipline." Thank you, God, for your discipline, as it is our gateway to knowledge and divine connection to you. Lord, I honor you today and forever.

In Jesus' name,

Amen

Reflection: In what area of your life do you desire for God to remove temptation and increase discipline?

Serve In a Spirit of Love

*Praise the Lord; praise God our savior!
For each day he carries us in his arms.*
PSALMS 68:19 (NLT)

Dear Gracious Heavenly Father,

Thank you for blessing me with such a beautiful village. Currently in my life, there has been a lot of change in a short period of time. I have had to be flexible, remain humble, stay focused and most importantly, have faith in you. Life is not void of difficulties that challenge me and that is why I am so grateful for your love. In Psalms 68:19, your Word says:

"Praise the Lord; praise God our savior! For each day He carries us in His arms." I know you are the real God! You show up in my life in amazing ways! In my devotional time with you, you confirmed that having a calm confidence in Christ is not arrogance. It is actually a spirit of humility that helps me to honor the God-given space that I occupy in this world. In doing so, you have allowed me to serve and be an authentic gift to others. Through your Holy Spirit, I am able to freely care for and love those around me. Thank you for living in my heart and soul. I will forever worship your Holy Name.

In Jesus' name,

Amen

> *Reflection: How has your relationship with serving God impacted the other relationships in your life? I believe your vibe attracts your tribe. Today, take a moment to acknowledge and pray for those supportive individuals in your village.*

SERVITUDE, LEADERSHIP & WISDOM

A Servant's Heart

> But when you give to the needy, do not let your
> left hand know what your right hand is doing.
> MATTHEW 6:3 (NLT)

Dear Gracious Heavenly Father,

Thank you for your unconditional love, mercy and grace. I thank you for being raised by a mother who knew how important it was to have a relationship with you and understand your word. In Matthew 6:3, you taught us:

"But when you give to the needy, do not let your left hand know what your right hand is doing." Father, you want us to be generous in an intrinsic way, to develop a desire to give from the heart, not to receive accolades from men, because our reward is with you in heaven. When we give, help us to just do it with love and a kind heart. Thank you for being the best example of generosity and kindness. Help us to show love to one another without looking for anything in return because we know you are omnipotent and omniscient.

You know and see it all. Please continue to strengthen, cover and bless us all so that we may glorify you.

In Jesus' name,

Amen

Reflection: Why does a leader need to have a servant's heart?

Lessons Learned From God

> Keep putting into practice all you learned and received from me—everything you heard from me and saw me doing, then the God of peace will be with you.
>
> PHILIPPIANS 4:9 (NLT)

Dear Gracious Heavenly Father,

It's an honor to be your child and be a part of this royal family. My heart is filled with joy knowing that I am loved by you unconditionally. You have watched my rise and fall, only to catch me and place me back on the path that you have set for me. Father, I desire to be used as your spirit-filled vessel in amazing ways to uplift others for your glory. In Philippians 4:9, you teach us to:

"Keep putting into practice all you learned and received from me—everything you heard from me and saw me doing, then the God of peace will be with you." Each day as I grow closer to you, I pray that your light is reflected in the ways that I serve. Help me to demonstrate and implement what I have learned from your example into the work that I do. Increase my authenticity for the building of your kingdom. I humble myself before you today and give you thanks.

In Jesus' name,

Amen

Reflection: What is the most important lesson that God wants us to learn if we desire to serve him?

SERVITUDE, LEADERSHIP & WISDOM

Choose Today Whom You Will Serve

As for me and my household, we will serve the Lord.
JOSHUA **24:15** (NIV)

Dear Gracious Heavenly Father,

This is the day that you have made, we shall rejoice and be glad in it. Father, there are many different things surrounding us in our daily lives that can become a distraction from our true purpose. Our purpose is to serve and glorify you. I thank you for your word because you said:

"But if you refuse to serve the Lord, then choose today whom you will serve. Would you prefer the gods your ancestors served beyond the Euphrates? Or will it be the gods of the Amorites in whose land you now live? But as for me and my family, we will serve the Lord." (Joshua 24:15 NLT) I made a choice to serve you because I know in you there is peace, hope and renewal. Help me, Father, to keep you first in my life and follow the path that you have set for me. Thank you for your continued provision for my family. We worship you and give you praise.

In Jesus' name,

Amen

Reflection: How will you serve God along your journey?

Be Kind to One Another and Show Compassion

> For you have been called to live in freedom, my brothers and sisters. But don't use your freedom to satisfy your sinful nature. Instead, use your freedom to serve one another in love.
> GALATIANS 5:13 (NLT)

Dear Gracious Heavenly Father,

I give you praise, honor and glory, for you are so mighty. You are omnipotent and you hold this entire world in your hands. As we go about our day, please help us to remember to be kind to one another, show compassion and love as you have done for us time and time again. You desire for us to not only think of ourselves but to also think of others and ways that we can be of service. Thank you for giving us the opportunity to get to know you for ourselves because it is a sweet experience. Please continue to watch over us and keep everyone safe from harm. Send your angels to encamp all around us. We love you, Lord, and give you all the glory.

In Jesus' name,

Amen

Reflection: God shows his compassion for us in many ways. Select one special person in your life and show them compassion by providing a service. What will the service be?

More Like Jesus

Blessed are the pure in heart, for they will see God.
MATTHEW 5:8 (KJV)

Dear Gracious Heavenly Father,

Thank you for creating us in your likeness and image. There are so many important lessons in your word that teach us about having a heart for you. Just as Solomon told us in Proverbs 4:23, to guard our hearts and Psalms 51:10, reads: *"Create in me a clean heart, O God, and renew a steadfast spirit within me."*

Finally, Matthew 5:8 says, *"Blessed are the pure in heart, for they will see God."* I often think about how I need renewed strength to maintain a pure heart if I truly desire to serve you. Along with receiving the gift of salvation, we need a new heart, which is what you promise to those who seek you for it. David had a willing spirit and a pure heart for you, Father, because he had a desire to serve. Help us to have pure intentions that flow from our hearts and manifest into actionable, deeds of positive impact in the world around us. Let us be reminded to whom we belong because we are your children. We honor you today and always.

In Jesus' name,

Amen

Reflection: Think of one actionable step that you can take today to demonstrate the positive impact that you desire to have in the world around you.

Persevere Despite Persecution

> "But I say to you who hear: Love your enemies, do good to those who hate you, bless those who curse you, and pray for those who spitefully use you."
> LUKE 6:27-28 (KJV)

Dear Heavenly Father,

Thank you for your presence in my life. Thank you for being my refuge and strength. Sometimes in this life, we will be mistreated or disrespected even when we are trying to do the right thing. Father, this can be so draining for the spirit so I ask that you give me strength, wisdom, patience and the courage to persevere. Ultimately, I want to glorify you because in your word you teach us that although we are eager to do good, evil is also present. Help me to continue to look to you for guidance and strength so that my focus remains on what is most important. Please continue to bless every individual across the globe who has been touched by the Angel Network. We magnify you today, for you are our King!

In Jesus' name,

Amen

Reflection: What will you ask God to help you focus on today, despite unpleasant interactions? How will you be proactive about maintaining your peace?

Guard Your Heart

> Guard your heart above all else, for it determines the course of your life.
> PROVERBS 4:23 (NLT)

Dear Gracious Heavenly Father,

I come before you today thanking you for your unconditional love and protection. Thank you for being so patient with me and for teaching me to listen for your voice and wisdom. Father, as we travel along life's journey, there may be times when "excess noise" from the environment clouds our judgment or we get discouraged by disappointments. There may even be times when we are exposed to lots of negativity. You have taught us in your word to guard our hearts above all else. Today, Father, help us to practice guarding our hearts by making strategic decisions about what we watch, listen to and read. Help us to saturate ourselves in your word so that we may be fortified in you. I thank you for your mercy and grace. I give you praise, honor and glory for all things.

In Jesus' name,

Amen

Reflection: Click below to view my YouTube video: "How's Your Diet?" What are you exposing yourself to on a regular basis and how does it serve you?
https://youtu.be/VlBv32dvIgQ

Be a Beacon of Light

Let your conversation be gracious and attractive so that you will have the right response for everyone.
COLOSSIANS 4:6 (NLT)

Dear Heavenly Father,

Thank you for giving us wisdom to know when to speak, when to be silent and when we should just listen. Sometimes our friends and family members just need a listening ear; someone that they can share their thoughts and feelings with, without feeling judged. When we walk closer to you, there should be evidence that you abide in our heart and soul. Father, help me to shine your light, be of comfort and speak life to those who cross my path. Help me to uplift and encourage others. In your word, you taught us to:

"Let our conversation be gracious and attractive so that we will have the right response for everyone." So, Father, thank you for teaching us the way to be a beacon of light in this world.

In Jesus' name,

Amen

Reflection: Reflect about your relationships. Ask God to give you wisdom in order to interact with others in healthy ways. Practice applying my P.T.R.L. (Pray, Think then Respond with Love) strategy to a situation that may currently be challenging for you.

Loyalty in Friendships

A friend is always loyal, and a brother is born to help in time of need.
PROVERBS 11:17

Dear Gracious Heavenly Father,

Thank you for the special individuals in my village that I have chosen to be my friends. They are loyal and understand the true meaning of friendship. In Proverbs 11:17, you taught us that:

"A friend is always loyal, and a brother is born to help in time of need." It is so important to have individuals in our lives that we can count on especially, in our time of need. My mother always taught us two are better than one. Father, help me to show those in my life how much I value our friendship and give me the wisdom to maintain those relationships in a healthy way. Thank you for your guidance.

In Jesus' name,

Amen

Reflection: In your journal, make a list of all the qualities about yourself. Choose 3 qualities and write: "I am" before the words. You have just created an affirmation. For example, I believe I am brave, therefore, I will write: I am brave and post it up where I can see it each day.

Grace From Above

> Blessed is the man who does not walk in the counsel
> of the wicked or stand in the way of sinners or sit in
> the seat of mockers. But his delight is in the law of the
> LORD, and on his law he meditates day and night.
> PSALMS 1:1 (NIV)

Dear Gracious Heavenly Father,

Thank you for the roof over my head, the clothes I wear, the shoes on my feet and the food I eat. Thank you for your mercy and grace. Thank you for the peace in my home and the wisdom to know when to just stay prayerful and listen. Your direction is needed because it serves as protection. Thank you for all the ways that you have blessed my family and me. I am grateful for every answered prayer. Please keep them as they travel. Continue to be our guide as we look to you. We bless your name forever.

In Jesus' name,

Amen

Reflection: Think about the ways that God protects you each day. What is an example of his grace in your life?

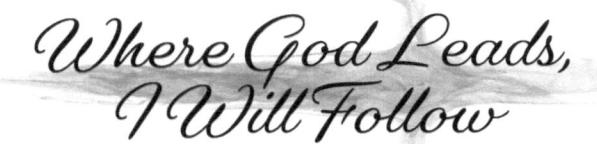

Where God Leads, I Will Follow

Train up a child in the way that he should go and when he is old, he will not depart from it.
PROVERBS 22:6 (KJV)

A Personal Prayer from the Author

Dear Gracious Heavenly Father,

Thank you for your wisdom and for life lessons in your Word that are so important for our growth and well being. For many years, Father, I prayed for my nephew and I asked you to send him to me, however, at the time it was not in your plan. Although, from my perspective, I may have viewed the events of life at the time as "falling apart;" you being omniscient knew that they were all falling into place. Today, you have given me the assignment of Auntie-Momma in my nephew's life and as I pour into him your word, I ask that you strengthen and fortify me. I also ask, Father, that your word not return void. I pray that it is planted on fertile soil because you taught us to:

"Direct our children onto the right path, and when they are older, they will not leave it." I see your hand over my nephew's life and hear evidence of you living in his heart as he prays each day. Please bless all the children in our village to have a desire to live a life that glorifies you and speaks to how they were taught by your word. We are so blessed to be your children. We love you, Lord! Help us to continue to look to you for guidance.

In Jesus' name,

Amen

> *Reflection: In what areas of your life do you need God to give you guidance and fortify you?*

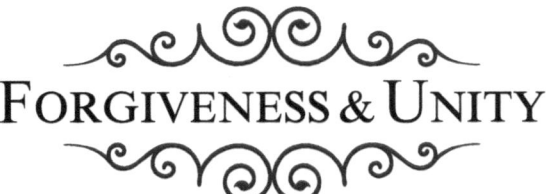

Forgiveness & Unity

Forgive Yourself

Open rebuke is better than secret love.
Proverbs 27:5 (KJV)

Dear Gracious Heavenly Father,

Thank you for my village that is made up of beautiful individuals which you have chosen to be in my life. In Proverbs 27:5, you have taught us that:

"Open rebuke is better than secret love." Thank you for teaching us through your Word how to approach confrontation in our relationships in healthy ways.

I remember when I was younger, my mother would always say, "If you have something against your brother about something done directly to you, bring it to your brother." My mother was teaching us how to be vulnerable and have those courageous conversations in order to maintain and nurture the relationships that are most important to us. Thank you, Father, for blessing us with such a wise mother who taught us to speak one on one with a person rather than gossip about being mistreated by them. Only you, Father, sit in the seat of judgment, so please give me the strength to forgive, the courage to confront and the patience to love in difficult times. Thank you for your precious word and guidance. I love you Lord.

In Jesus name,

Amen

> *Reflection: Take some quiet time to meditate and forgive yourself first before you ask the forgiveness of others.*

FORGIVENESS & UNITY

Forgive One Another

And be ye kind one to another, tenderhearted, forgiving one another, even as God for Christ's sake hath forgiven you.
EPHESIANS 4:32 (KJV)

Dear Precious Heavenly Father,

One of the most important commandments that we must follow is to love you and others. We must show love in the same way that you have shown love to us. At times, we will find ourselves in situations that may cause hurt and pain and in these moments finding the strength to forgive can be difficult. We need God's help to do so. Forgiveness is not for other people. It is for us. It allows our hearts to be pure and our minds to be clear in order to focus on treating others with dignity and respect. With this mindset, we can apply Ephesians 4:32 to our daily walk with Christ as it reads, *"And be ye kind one to another, tenderhearted, forgiving one another, even as God for Christ's sake hath forgiven you."* Thank you for your unconditional love, Father, and for being patient with us as we learn to truly forgive ourselves and others. We love you for first loving us.

In Jesus' name,

Amen

Reflection: Try writing a letter to the individual/s from whom you seek forgiveness. Pray before you send the letter and know that God is always watching over you. He always forgives.

Love Your Enemies!

"Love your enemies! Do good to them.
LUKE 6:35 (NLT)

Dear Gracious Heavenly Father,

In Luke Chapter 6:35, you tell us to:

"Love your enemies! Do good to them. Lend to them without expecting to be repaid. Then your reward from heaven will be very great, and you will truly be acting as children of the Most High, for he is kind to those who are unthankful and wicked."

It is so easy to love those who are kind, thoughtful and gentle towards us. When it comes to someone that has hurt us or disrespected us, loving them is the real challenge. So, Father, I ask that you give me a teachable spirit, one that is pleasing to you and follows after your heart. Strengthen me in times of frustration (when I feel forsaken by others who may have mistreated me) and allow me to be comforted by your unconditional love. Heal and restore relationships today as only you can Father. We ask these things in your precious name and give you thanks.

In Jesus' name,

Amen

Reflection: Ask God to help you forgive those who have trespassed against you so that you may worship Him with a pure heart.

FORGIVENESS & UNITY

Fully Forgive Others

Love means doing what God has commanded us, and he has commanded us to love one another, just as you heard from the beginning.
2 JOHN 1:6 (NLT)

Dear Precious Heavenly Father,

Thank you for demonstrating what true love is so that we are able to look to you and follow your commandments. 2 John 1:6 explains that:

"Love means doing what God has commanded us, and he has commanded us to love one another, just as you heard from the beginning." Father, please help us to first, truly forgive, so that we can genuinely love with a pure heart. Love is patient. Love is kind. Love will never abandon us. When we truly love, touch our hearts to be free from the bondage of holding grudges against one another. Strengthen us to rise above and be the beacon of light and love that you have always been to us. We give you praise, honor and glory forever.

In Jesus' name,

Amen

Reflection: Ask God to purify your heart so that you are able to fully forgive individuals and maintain peace in your life.

Mold Me, Jesus!

> *May God, who gives this patience and encouragement, help you live in complete harmony with each other, as is fitting for followers of Christ Jesus.*
> ROMANS 15:5 (NLT)

Dear Gracious Heavenly Father,

You are our Messiah! You exemplify patience, faithfulness and love. Help me to surrender to your guidance and be still to know that you are God so that I may move only when you speak. Mold me in your image to live harmoniously in fellowship with others as you have ordained. Thank you for your love and kindness. I glorify your name forever.

In Jesus' name,

Amen

Reflection: When you create your things "to-do" list or review your week at a glance, take a moment and thank God in advance for his guidance and favor over your life as you complete your tasks.

A Prayer For Our Nation

A Unified Focus For the Kingdom of God

"For where two or three gather together as my followers, I am there among them."
Matthew 18:20 (NIV)

A Personal Prayer from the Author

Dear Precious Heavenly Father,

I come before you today with a grateful and humble heart. I thank you for inspiring me to bring together beautiful women of God who desire to worship you and fellowship together. A dear friend shared a word with me from Matthew 18:20 about my new assignment. The Thriving, Encouraging and Authentic (T.E.A. Room) a monthly gathering was created. She reminded me that you have reassured us, *"For where two or three gather together as my followers, I am there among them."*

Thank you for confirming your Word and helping me to truly experience your presence; whether that is in a large congregation or with two or three are gathered in your name. It is an honor to unite and glorify you. My prayer for our people is that we continue to come together and demonstrate a genuine love for one another that produces a unified focus on the kingdom agenda by uplifting others. May you bring peace to our nation and families. We love you Lord and glorify your name forever.

In Jesus' name,

Amen

Reflection: Where do you believe unity begins and how do we cultivate it in healthy ways?

A Prayer For Our Nation

Dear Gracious Heavenly Father,

I come before you today with a humble, yet heavy heart. Our world needs you. Our world is crying out for leadership, guidance, love, compassion and unity. In your Word, you told us that we may become angry but don't sin because vengeance is yours. My heart is heavy today for my own personal loss of missing my parents and also our grieving nation. We are in need of healing and I pray today for every family across the nation whose heart is hurting right now. Father, you are our healer, our Jehovah Rapha. Please allow us to open our hearts and minds to stand up for what is right and help us to make our world a better place. We believe in your ability to heal and restore the hearts of your people. Give us peace that surpasses all understanding as we pull closer together.

In Jesus' name,

Amen

Notes

www.ingramcontent.com/pod-product-compliance
Lightning Source LLC
Chambersburg PA
CBHW030154100526
44592CB00009B/276